G 79

SEQUENTIAL MEDICAL TRIALS

SEQUENTIAL
MEDICAL TRIALS

by

P. ARMITAGE
M.A., PH.D.

*Statistical Research Unit of the Medical Research Council,
London School of Hygiene and Tropical Medicine*

BLACKWELL
SCIENTIFIC PUBLICATIONS
OXFORD

First printed November 1960

PRINTED IN GREAT BRITAIN BY ADLARD & SON LTD
BARTHOLOMEW PRESS, DORKING

PREFACE

It is now widely accepted that the most reliable way to compare the effectiveness of alternative medical treatments is to carry out a controlled trial, in which the treatments are allocated at random. In recent years a number of these clinical trials have been conducted by sequential methods, and there appears to be a growing interest in this development. In a sequential analysis the observations are examined as they become available, and the total number of subjects to enter the trial is not predetermined, but depends on the accumulating results.

Sequential analysis has an immediate appeal in clinical research. Patients normally enter an investigation serially and a continuous scrutiny of the results is usually quite feasible. Rather more important is the ethical consideration, which requires that any unnecessary use of inferior treatments should be avoided. The investigator will, therefore, frequently wish to bring a trial to an early close if an important difference can, at that early stage, be established.

The present time seems a suitable moment to attempt a general survey of this topic. There are now a sufficient number of examples of medical trials conducted by sequential analysis to show that the methods are practicable. Unfortunately, the basic information about these methods has been scattered through the statistical and medical literature, and the few expository papers are neither comprehensive nor up-to-date.

I have attempted in this book to write an account of the principles underlying the subject, and to provide sufficient detail about the methods to enable the medical practitioner to proceed without necessarily feeling obliged to consult a statistician. Most of the techniques are simple, and are conveniently carried out by plotting points on charts. I have omitted as much mathematics from the text as possible.

The first chapter contains an account of the main statistical concepts used in the book, but this account is too brief to serve as much more than an *aide-mémoire*. The reader who is entirely unfamiliar with the basic concepts of probability, significance tests, etc. would be well advised to read one of the many elementary books on the subject. At a first reading one or two sections of the book may seem rather more complicated than the rest, and may easily be skipped. Chapter 7 will probably give the most trouble.

Although mathematical proofs are not included in the book, I have tried to give adequate references to the relevant publications. For the benefit of the statistician, I have included an Appendix, in which some points are discussed which are not covered satisfactorily in the literature. I hope this book will interest statisticians working outside the medical field. The methods described here were evolved for a particular type of problem encountered in medical research, but I think it is quite possible that they may find other fields of application; in industry, for example.

I am grateful to the National Bureau of Standards for permission to print (in Table 6.1) extracts from their publication *Tables to facilitate sequential t-tests*. Various parts of the manuscripts were read by Dr G. E. Bartsch, Dr D. R. Cox, Professor A. Bradford Hill, Mr M. A. Schneiderman and Dr H. M. Schoolman, and I have benefited by their criticisms. The more felicitous passages in the book may safely be ascribed to them: for the others I alone am to blame. I am most grateful to Miss Irene Allen for computational help and for typing the manuscript; and to Mrs B. M. Hunt for preparing the diagrams for the press.

June, 1960   P. ARMITAGE

CONTENTS

CHAPTER ONE

MEDICAL TRIALS

1.1. Introduction

There has been, since the early 1940's, an increasing use of controlled medical trials to compare the effectiveness of different therapeutic or prophylactic treatments. This book is concerned with a particular aspect of controlled trials, namely the use of sequential methods of design and analysis, by means of which the results of a trial can be examined continuously as they become available and can thus form the basis of a decision to stop the trial at a suitable point. In Chapter 2 (and, briefly, at the end of the present chapter) we shall discuss the nature of sequential experimentation, and the reasons for considering sequential methods in this particular field of investigation. The later chapters present detailed methods appropriate for various circumstances and discuss some of the difficulties which may arise in practice.

Before considering the sequential aspects of our subject it is perhaps appropriate to discuss the principles of controlled trials in general. This chapter forms an introduction to the rest of the book, and the opportunity will be taken to summarize some of the statistical considerations involved in this type of study. There are a number of publications about controlled trials, for instance Hill (1951, 1956, 1960) and Witts (1959), which deal more fully with many aspects of the subject than does this brief survey, particularly from the medical and practical points of view. The reader unacquainted with elementary statistical concepts would be well advised to consult a standard book on the subject, as for example Hill (1956), Moroney (1956) or Bailey (1959).

1.2. Comparative experimentation

If the same medical treatment is given to a number of patients with the same illness, their apparent responses will inevitably differ. Similar variation in response will appear if the treatment is given repeatedly to the same patient. Any attempt to compare the relative effectiveness of two or more treatments must therefore take into account the unpredictable variation in response from one occasion to another. The problem presents itself in almost every field of biological experimentation, for it is in the nature of biological material to show some degree of unpredictable variability.

It is standard practice in experimental biology to make *simultaneous* comparisons of treatments, for if the treatments are applied at different times any apparent difference in response may be due not to the treatments themselves but to some change in the environment, in the observer, or in the experimental units to which the treatments are applied. In clinical experimentation, retrospective comparisons are particularly hazardous. If the results of applying a certain treatment to a group of patients are compared with those obtained in the previous year or two with another treatment, we can never be sure that the comparison is not seriously affected by some difference in the composition of the groups. For instance, the groups may differ in the proportion of severe cases, or in the proportion of patients who have failed to respond to previous treatment. There may also have been changes in the standards of diagnosis, or in some environmental factor which may affect the response. It is perhaps even more dangerous to compare groups of patients treated in different centres, for in this sort of comparison differences in the type of patient entering the two series are almost unavoidable.

If it is accepted that a reliable comparative experiment must involve the simultaneous use of the treatments under study, the question then arises how this should be carried out. A comparison, within the same centre, at the same time, of patients who happen to have been given the different treatments, is quite unreliable. The patients have probably been given different treatments by their physicians because they differed to some extent in the nature or severity of their disease, and such variation may suffice to explain any difference (or lack of difference) in response which may be observed. A comparison of various occasions on which different treatments happen to have been used on the same patient is open to a similar objection. The need is for some method of ensuring that the groups of experimental units (in this case different subjects or different occasions on the same subject) which are allocated to different treatments are free from any possible systematic bias.

It has been generally recognized, since the work of R. A. (now Sir Ronald) Fisher in agricultural research in the 1920's, that a valid comparison can be achieved only by some form of randomization. The experimental units (which, in the type of trial referred to above will be different patients) should be allocated either completely at random, or with an element of randomization, to the groups which will receive various treatments. The word 'randomization' and the phrase 'at random' imply some chance mechanism such as tossing a coin, but experimental workers can, as it were, toss their coins vicariously by using tables of random sampling numbers (for instance, those of Fisher and Yates (1957) or Hill (1956)). Instructions for using these tables will be found elsewhere and will not be given in full detail here. In many clinical trials patients enter the study serially, and this may afford an opportunity to use some effective and adequate substitute for strict randomization, such as allocation by the last digit of the hospital number. Whatever method of randomization is used, it is advisable that a patient should be entered into the trial *before* the randomization list is consulted. If the physician knows initially which treatment a patient would have, he may be biased in deciding whether or not to enter this patient into the trial. This bias may cause a serious deficiency of particular types of patient in some of the treatment groups. A discussion of methods of randomization for sequential trials is contained in §2.5.

1.3. The problem of medical experimentation

Since the 1939–45 war many medical trials, controlled by randomization, have been carried out. In clinical medicine these range from small-scale investigations under the control of one doctor to large-scale studies requiring the co-operation of many doctors and institutions. Examples of the latter are the series of clinical trials of different treatments for pulmonary tuberculosis conducted by the Medical Research Council (for example, M.R.C., 1948, 1955), and the series of clinical trials in cancer chemotherapy performed under the auspices of the U.S. Public Health Service (Endicott, 1957). In preventive medicine, where attack rates are normally fairly low, the requisite large numbers of observations can usually be made only by co-operative effort. Examples in this field are the M.R.C. trials of vaccines against whooping cough (M.R.C., 1959) and tuberculosis (M.R.C., 1956) and the trials of poliomyelitis vaccine in the United States (Poliomyelitis Vaccine Evaluation Center, 1955) and in this country (M.R.C., 1957). It is a matter of established fact, then, that controlled medical trials can be successfully organized and can provide useful information.

There are, however, well-known ethical difficulties which may prevent the carrying out of a trial which would otherwise have provided valuable information. A doctor who believes that one of the treatments under consideration is more effective than another cannot commit patients under his care to the treatment he believes to be inferior. Frequently, however, there will be no convincing evidence as to the relative merits of the rival treatments. It is then generally felt to be no more unethical to treat some patients by each method than to use one treatment throughout. It has, indeed, been argued that the doctor is under a moral obligation to use the available treatments in such a way that he acquires information about their relative merits as quickly and effectively as possible. The ethical problems in sequential trials are no greater, and, as we shall see below, may be less, than in the more established type of randomized trial, and it is hardly necessary to elaborate them further here. For further discussion see Hill (1956).

1.4. Experimental design

In many branches of science and technology, particularly agricultural and industrial research, the design of comparative experiments has reached a high degree of complexity. Techniques are available for making the most efficient use of a limited amount of experimental material, in investigating the combined effects of many different factors. The book by Cox (1958a) provides a clear account of the principles underlying the various types of design which are now available, and further details are contained in the book by Cochran and Cox (1957).

In medical trials hitherto, relatively simple designs have usually been employed. The main reason is probably that an experimental investigation undertaken in the clinic or the hospital ward is difficult enough to plan and carry out, even with the simplest of experimental designs. Further elaboration may be prohibitive. However, as the randomized trial becomes more and more firmly established and clinical workers become more familiar with the practical problems, it should be possible to use more complex designs. Clinical responses are influenced by many factors, and experimental designs which investigate their effects and eliminate them from the treatment comparisons which are the principal object of interest, should be valuable.

In this book we shall consider only single-factor designs, i.e. designs to compare the comparative effects of a single set of treatments, as distinct from factorial designs in which combinations of two or more sets of treatments are used. It is useful to make a broad distinction between two types of design — those by which each subject has only one of the alternative treatments, so that treatment comparisons are made *between* subjects; and those by which each subject has more than one treatment, so that comparisons are made *within* subjects. Within-subject comparisons are most naturally made in studies of chronic disease, where a relatively short-term relief is sought. Comparisons between subjects are usually inevitable for acute diseases where the available treatment periods are limited, but may also be necessary in some studies of chronic disease where a particular treatment has to be applied over a long period of time, or where a long interval must elapse between the start of treatment and the evaluation of response. Prophylactic trials, which normally involve rather long follow-up studies, also fall naturally into the between-patient category.

On the whole, we should expect to achieve greater precision by making comparisons within, rather than between, subjects. For, by doing so, we eliminate the variation in response from one subject to another. There is, however, the possibility (observed by Meier *et al.* (1958)) that if the treatment period were extended sufficiently to enable more than one treatment to be used on each subject, any differences between the effects of the treatments might gradually diminish. This dilution of the treatment comparisons might outweigh any reduction in variability, in which case it would be better to make comparisons between subjects on the basis of the initial course of treatment. Another difficulty which may arise in a within-patient trial is that if the courses of treatment follow each other too closely, the effect of one treatment may carry over to the next period, when a different treatment is being applied.

If the response observed during a treatment period depends strongly on which position in the series it occupies (for example, whether it is the first, second or third of a series of three courses of treatment), it may be useful to arrange the order in a systematic way, as for instance in a latin square arrangement (Cochran and Cox, 1957, section 4.3). In this book, however, we shall assume that when various treatments are applied to the same subject their order is determined by random choice.

In experiments involving between-subject comparisons, some degree of reduction in the random variation may be achieved by grouping together subjects whose response might be expected to be similar (say, for reasons of age, sex, or severity of the disease). These groups are technically known as '*blocks*'. Treatments may then be compared from the responses *within* each of the blocks. In agricultural experiments it is usually simple to arrange that in each block every treatment is applied equally frequently. But in a clinical trial, for which patients become available serially in time, such absolute symmetry would be difficult to achieve, and is hardly worth striving for. If patients are allocated to treatments at random, with no regard for any stratification by age, sex and so on, the results can always be examined at the end to see whether these factors appear to have any appreciable effect, and if so the analysis can take this into account. There is, however, some advantage in arranging that in any one stratum the numbers allocated to different treatments are always nearly equal, and that at certain points (for instance, after each successive group of ten patients has entered this stratum) they are exactly equal. For further details see §2.5.

In a sequential analysis the problem is a little more pressing, in that we have to decide whether the continuous scrutiny of the results shall take into account any stratification of the population. As will be explained in §2.5, many of the available methods of sequential analysis are conveniently performed on *pairs* of observations, one member of each pair being allocated at random to each of two treatments. This pairing may be entirely at random, no regard being paid to strata. Alternatively, if one is fairly confident that some factors – like age, sex or severity – appreciably affect the response, these factors should be used to define strata, and successive patients falling within the same stratum may then be paired. Excessive stratification should not be undertaken lightly, though, for at any stage of the enquiry there will be an appreciable number of unpaired subjects — all falling into different strata, and this wastage may counterbalance any possible increase in precision over that achieved by unstratified pairing.

Pairing of successive entrants to a trial, with or without stratification, automatically removes one possible source of variation — a gradual trend in response throughout the trial, affecting both treatment groups equally. Such a trend may occur for environmental reasons, or because either the standard of assessment of response or the nature of the disease in different patients is gradually changing. Whatever the reason for it, such a time trend would hardly affect a comparison of responses for two patients entering the trial at almost the same time, and the precision of the final comparison is thereby increased.

1.5. Statistical analysis: tests, decisions and estimates

Because of the variability of biological responses, any conclusion drawn from a comparative experiment is subject to some degree of uncertainty. It *may* happen that in the random allocation of patients to two treatment groups, those who are more resistant to treatment have fallen preponderantly into one, rather than the other, group. It is possible, but unlikely. The methods of statistics enable the experimenter to assess the extent to which his results are likely to have been influenced by random variation.

Suppose that, in a randomized medical trial, two treatments, A and B, are to be compared. At the end of the trial we may wish to compare their effects on various criteria of response. For each of these criteria we shall normally wish to draw one of the three following conclusions:

(a) A is preferable to B;
(a)' B is preferable to A;
(b) the evidence before us is inadequate to allow us to decide between A and B.

Another way of putting this is to say that we wish to make one of three decisions, namely to act as though (a) A were the better treatment; (a)' B were the better; or (b) A and B were about equally effective.

We should naturally like to conclude (a) or (a)' only when there is reasonably good evidence that a difference really exists. More than one way of expressing this requirement quantitatively has been proposed, but the approach which we shall adopt is the conventional one based on *significance tests*. We can arrange that if A and B were equally effective (a supposition called the *null hypothesis*), then in a series of repetitions of the experiment we should be led to the erroneous conclusions (a) or (a)' only a small proportion of the time. Suppose these proportions are a and a'. We can express the situation in different words by saying that on the null hypothesis the probabilities of reaching the erroneous conclusions (a) and (a)' are, respectively, a and a'. It is customary to say that results leading to (a) or (a)' are *significant at the $a + a'$ level in a two-sided test*. We shall normally consider procedures for which $a = a'$ (i.e. $a + a' = 2a$) and refer to them as *two-sided* tests at the $2a$ significance level. The significance level is often expressed as a percentage. Thus, if $a = 0·025$, we might refer to the two-sided 5 per cent. significance level.

The results which are labelled 'significant' will be those which in some sense deviate to the greatest extent from the results expected on the null hypothesis. An example may make this clear. Suppose that, in a comparative trial of two analgesic agents, A and B, a number of patients requiring pain relief are each given A and B on two different occasions, the order of administration being randomly determined. They are then asked to express a preference for one or the other drug. Suppose that, of 30 patients willing to state a preference, 22 preferred A and 8 preferred B. Now, on the null hypothesis a preference for A is just as likely to be expressed as a preference for B; i.e. the probability that an expressed preference is for A rather than for B is $\frac{1}{2}$. Some straight-forward calculations in probability theory (using the *binomial* distribution) show that on the null hypothesis the probabilities of observing $0, 1, 2, \ldots, 30$, preferences for A, out of 30, are as shown in Table 1.1. Accumulating the probabilities from the most extreme values of x (0 and 30), towards the middle of the distribution, until the total just falls short of $0 \cdot 05$, we find that 0–9 and 21–30 each account for a probability of 0.021, making a total of $0 \cdot 042$. If any of these results occurred, they would be said to contradict the null hypothesis at the 5 per cent. significance level. The result actually found ($x = 22$) falls into this class. The probability of obtaining a result at least as extreme as that observed (i.e. $x = 22$–30, or 0–8) is $0 \cdot 016$, and the observed

Table 1. 1. Binomial distribution of the number of preferences, out of 30, in favour of treatment A, on the null hypothesis that both types of preference are equally likely.

Number of preferences, x, in favour of A	Probability	Cumulative probability	
		From $x = 0$	From $x = 30$
0	0·000	0·000	..
1	0·000	0·000	..
2	0·000	0·000	..
3	0·000	0·000	..
4	0·000	0·000	..
5	0·000	0·000	..
6	0·001	0·001	..
7	0·002	0·003	..
8	0·005	0·008	..
9	0·013	0·021	..
10	0·028	0·049	..
11	0·051	0·100	..
12	0·081	0·181	..
13	0·112	0·292	..
14	0·135	0·428	..
15	0·144	0·572	0·572
16	0·135	..	0·428
17	0·112	..	0·292
18	0·081	..	0·181
19	0·051	..	0·100
20	0·028	..	0·049
21	0·013	..	0·021
22	0·005	..	0·008
23	0·002	..	0·003
24	0·001	..	0·001
25	0·000	..	0·000
26	0·000	..	0·000
27	0·000	..	0·000
28	0·000	..	0·000
29	0·000	..	0·000
30	0·000	..	0·000
	1·000		

results may therefore be said to contradict the null hypothesis not only at the 5 per cent. level, but also at the 2 per cent. level ($0 \cdot 016$ being less than $0 \cdot 02$, or 2 per cent.). The probability of a result at least as extreme as that observed (in this example, $0 \cdot 016$) is frequently denoted by P, and serves to indicate the degree of significance at which the null hypothesis is contradicted.

The significance level at which the investigator will be willing to conclude (a) or (a)′ will depend on the special circumstances of the trial: if general experience and an examination of relevant evidence predispose the investigator to believe that a difference in a particular direction is likely, he will probably be willing to accept a moderate degree of significance, say the 5 per cent. level, as being adequate. If a difference in a particular direction seems highly unlikely on general grounds, then he may fail to be convinced by anything less than a high degree of significance — say, corresponding to the 1 per cent. or $0 \cdot 1$ per cent. level. The extreme situation is one in which differences in one direction only are considered to be possible; that is, we decline, under any circumstances, to draw conclusion (a)′. The significance test is then called *one-sided*. In the example above, for instance, if we contemplated only the possibility that A could be the preferable treatment, we should regard the results $x = 20$–30 as being significant at the one-sided 5 per cent. level, since the total probability of these values of x is $0 \cdot 049$, just less than $0 \cdot 05$. In my view one-sided significance tests are inappropriate in most, if not all, medical trials. Most of the preliminary evidence that can be brought to bear on a comparison under trial is only indirectly relevant, and one must be prepared for the possibility that the crucial clinical test may reverse all preconceived judgments. Even in a trial to compare the relative effects of an active drug and an inert placebo, the active drug may exhibit unsuspected ill-effects which make it the less effective treatment.

Frequently the result of a significance test will determine what action or decision the investigator takes about the future policy of treatment for the type of patient studied in the trial. There may, however, be a clear distinction between the conclusions drawn about the relative merits of the treatments, and the practical policy. For instance, even though the significance test is two-sided, allowing one of the three conclusions (a), (a)′ or (b) to be drawn, there may be two distinct courses of action — to recommend a new drug for future use, or not. Again, unsuspected side effects exhibited by a new drug may preclude its future use, even though the statistical analysis has shown that, on the criterion of improvement which was originally chosen, patients

2

clearly benefited by its use. A further distinction must be drawn between the policy decisions of the investigator, and those made by other doctors examining the same evidence. Their assessment of previous work in this field may differ from his, and they may feel that stronger evidence is required before they can be induced to abandon a well-tried treatment. Finally, even if a doctor is convinced that *some* improvement in response will be achieved by using a very expensive treatment, he may feel that the benefit is likely to be so slight that the extra expense would be unjustifiable, particularly for minor ailments.

This brings us to another aspect of statistical analysis — the estimation of the extent of the difference between the effects of various treatments. The exact procedure to be followed depends on the type of response used; for example, this may be the mean value of some measurement, or it may be the proportion of subjects showing a certain degree of improvement in a fixed period of time. We may postulate some 'true' difference between the means or between the proportions; that is, the difference which would be observed in an indefinitely long series of observations, showing the same sort of random variability as those actually made. Then standard methods are available for making an estimate of the true difference, and also for indicating the extent to which the estimate is likely to be in error owing to random variation. The usual procedure is to quote '*confidence limits*' for the true value, which have the property that the true value will be included within the limits a stated proportion of the time. For example, 95 per cent. confidence limits will include the true value 19 times out of 20; once in 20 times, on the average, the observed results will be so atypical of the long-run behaviour that the confidence limits exclude the true value.

1.6. The amount of experimentation

The more observations an experimenter makes, the more precise will be the treatment comparisons; that is, the smaller will be the extent to which the comparisons are influenced by random fluctuations. The extent to which the effects of two treatments differ may be measured by the difference between the mean values of some measurement of response in a very large series of observations. As in §1.5 we shall call this the 'true' difference. It may be that a small experiment would be insufficiently sensitive to detect this true difference, in the sense that the probability of obtaining a result which significantly contradicted the null hypothesis would be rather low. As the number of observations is increased, the probability that the observed difference is significant at a particular level, say the 2α level, will increase, and with a sufficiently large number of observations we can make this probability as high as we please. The probability of obtaining a result significant at some chosen level, is called the *power* of a test. It depends, of course, on the value of the true difference. For a given size of experiment, the bigger the true difference the greater will be the power.

Consider the binomial significance test described in the last section, for an experiment providing 30 preferences. As a measure of the 'true'

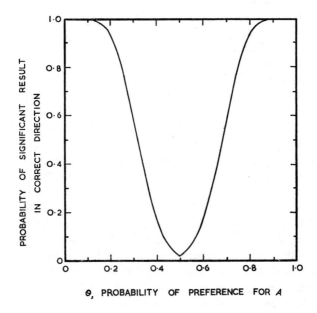

Fig. 1.1. Power curve for two-sided test at the 5 per cent. level, in a series of 30 binomial preferences. θ is the probability of a preference for treatment A, and the null hypothesis is that $\theta = \frac{1}{2}$.

difference, we can conveniently use the probability that a preference is expressed for A rather than B. This quantity, denoted by θ, is the proportion of A preferences in an indefinitely long series. We have seen that the results $x = 0$–9 or 21–30 significantly contradict the null hypothesis at the 5 per cent. level. Fig. 1.1 shows the power of the test for different values of θ. The vertical scale represents the probability of obtaining a result which significantly contradicts the null hypothesis *in the correct direction*. The power is low for values of θ near $\frac{1}{2}$, but rises as θ approaches 0 or 1. A larger experiment would have a power curve which rose more steeply as θ departed from $\frac{1}{2}$; for a smaller experiment the curve would be shallower.

A convenient way to specify the sensitivity of an experiment is to consider values of the true difference which can be detected with a fairly high power. We shall denote this high value of the power by $1 - \beta$. The probabilities α and β are thus both fairly small quantities, and are sometimes referred to as *errors of the first and second kinds*, respectively. In the experiment represented by Fig. 1.1, it can be calculated that if the probability of an A preference, θ, is as high as $0 \cdot 81$, then the probability is about $0 \cdot 95$ that the outcome of the experiment will be in the 5 per cent. significance zone. In other words, the experiment has a power of $1 - \beta = 0 \cdot 95$ with respect to the value $\theta = 0 \cdot 81$.

If the random variability to be encountered in the data were accurately known, one could envisage the size of an experiment being determined as follows. The experimenter would decide what value of the true difference was so important that he should allow himself a high chance $(1 - \beta)$ of detecting it at a particular significance level (2α) — if it really exists. Here α and β would be fairly low probabilities, say $0 \cdot 05$ or less. In practice, it might not be possible to estimate the random variability very accurately, and the choice of the critical value for the true difference, and of α and β, would be arbitrary. But at least it would be possible to devise a figure for the size of the experiment which satisfied some fairly reasonable requirements. It is rather common experience that figures derived in this way tend to be higher than had been bargained for by the experimenter! If so, he would have to revise his requirements, making, as it were, less demands of his experiment, until finally a compromise was reached between the conflicting aims of sensitivity and economy, tending respectively to enlarge and contract the experiment.

The power curve in Fig. 1.1 is symmetrical. We shall see in later chapters (§§2.3, 3.7) that sequential experimentation provides an opportunity to concentrate effort on the detection of differences in one particular direction. In these circumstances the power curve may rise much more steeply for departures from the null hypothesis in one direction than for those in the other direction.

1.7. The tendency to experiment sequentially

The statistical methods which have been briefly summarized above are applied a great deal in various fields of enquiry, and are fully elaborated and exemplified in many books on the subject. In almost all the 'classical' methods, the probabilities (such as α and β in the arguments used above) refer to imaginary repetitions of the experiment, with the number of observations kept constant. This restriction is natural if this number was predetermined as part of the experimental design, or if (as in most non-experimental work) it was a consequence of restrictions (such as amount of time available) *independent of the particular observations made.*

Medical trials, as we have seen, are characterized particularly by ethical difficulties, and it is quite natural that an investigator conducting a randomized trial should wish to follow the results closely, and continuously, as they become available, so that an important difference may be quickly detected and the trial brought to a close. The fact that observations in a medical trial are usually made serially encourages this sort of continuous scrutiny, and it seems likely that many trials performed in the past have been conducted in this way. Under these circumstances the probabilities associated with classical significance tests are no longer appropriate. The reason is not difficult to see. If we are continually on the look-out for a 'significant' difference there will be a higher probability of finding one purely by chance (in the absence of real treatment differences), than if the test were performed merely once, at the final stage of the trial.

Table 1. 2. Effect of repeated significance tests (two-sided 5 per cent. level) in an experiment in which preferences are recorded serially.

	Number of preferences, n					
	6	10	20	30	40	50
Probability, on null hypothesis, that "significant" result has been found at or before this stage	0·032	0·090	0·177	0·223	0·273	0·317

That this is more than a trivial difficulty may be seen from the probabilities given in Table 1.2. These refer to an experiment of the type described in §1.5. Suppose that, instead of analysing a fixed number of preferences, the investigator arranges that the subjects make their preferences serially, and after each new result he tests the null hypothesis at the 5 per cent. level. As soon as a 'significant' result is observed he stops the trial. The first stage at which it is possible to get a result significant at this level is after 6 preferences, the contrast being significant if all 6 preferences are in the same direction. Table 1.2 shows the probability that a 'significant' result will have been observed, and the trial stopped, before various numbers of preferences have been recorded.

These probabilities are calculated on the assumption that the null hypothesis is true. By the time 50 subjects have recorded their preferences, there is a chance of almost 1 in 3 that a 'significant' result will have been reported — even though the treatments are really equally effective. In fact, if the experiment continues indefinitely, the investigator is certain to get a 'significant' result eventually.

If the probabilities defining the significance level and the power are to be regarded as useful features of an analysis, we must seek some method of analysis which takes into account the sequential nature of the experimentation, and this in its turn requires that the conditions under which the trial is to be stopped at any stage shall be clearly defined. In the next chapter we consider the general nature of sequential experimentation, and some of its detailed features.

CHAPTER TWO

SEQUENTIAL EXPERIMENTATION

2.1. The nature of sequential experimentation

Experimentation may be broadly defined as 'sequential' if its conduct at any stage depends on the results so far obtained. In this sense almost any programme of experimentation is sequential, since the questions investigated in any particular experiment are usually influenced by previous work, and the results will to some extent determine the course of future research. The way in which programmes of research are carried out is difficult to describe in general quantitative terms, and more progress can be made if attention is confined to a group of closely related experiments of which the general strategy can be defined at the outset. Statisticians working in the chemical industry, for instance, have considered the problem of designing a series of experiments to estimate the conditions under which the yield of some chemical, produced by a particular manufacturing process, is as high as possible.

In this book we impose two further restrictions, by considering only *single* experiments (that is, single medical trials), and by permitting the results to influence only the number of observations made; we do not, for example, envisage the possibility that treatments are changed from time to time during the experiment. The section of statistical theory called *sequential analysis*, which is concerned almost entirely with this situation, is based largely on the work of the late A. Wald, whose book *Sequential analysis* (1947) should be consulted for mathematical details. The publication by the Statistical Research Group, Columbia University (1945) is a non-mathematical exposition of Wald's results. The use of sequential analysis in medical trials has been discussed generally by Bross (1952, 1958) and Armitage (1954, 1958b).

2.2. Reasons for sequential investigations

What are the purposes and advantages of sequential analysis? We note here three of the main reasons for conducting sequential investigations.

In any investigation, some of these aims may be subsidiary or entirely irrelevant, and the most appropriate sequential design will vary accordingly.

(a) *Economy*. There are a number of situations in which a large number of materials, or consignments of goods, have to be sorted into groups of differing quality, by means of a test the outcome of which is subject to some uncertainty. Examples are industrial sampling procedures, by which batches of manufactured items are accepted or rejected by the inspection of random samples; and procedures for the screening of drugs for a specific activity, by means of a biological test. Economy in testing can usually be achieved by performing more sampling or experimentation for some incoming materials than for others; the results themselves determine whether many, or a few, observations are required on any particular material. Since the test procedure is to be applied a large number of times, any reduction in the *average* length of a test, without any loss in the ability to distinguish between good and bad quality, will usually be welcome. If enough is known about the economics of the situation it may be possible to choose the rules of procedure so as to minimize, or at any rate reduce, the financial cost of the whole operation.

(b) *Estimation with desired accuracy*. We may wish to estimate some characteristic of a population – say, the mean urinary concentration of some substance in patients with a particular disease – to a specified level of accuracy. The precision of the estimate will depend not only on the sample size but also on the variability of the observations, and this may not be at all well known. The investigation may be carried out in two stages. A small pilot investigation will provide an estimate of the variability of the observations, and hence an indication of the number of observations needed in the second stage, to achieve the required accuracy. This process can be extended by allowing a series of more than two stages of sampling, but Anscombe (1954) has suggested that one could collect observations gradually, until the precision of the estimate (as measured by the customary formulae for standard errors) reaches the desired level. The essential point here is that the classical measure of precision informs us when approximately the required precision has been reached, *even though the sampling is sequential* (cf. §8.3).

(c) *Ethical consideration*. We have already noted in §1.7 that the organizer of a medical trial, anxious to avoid any unnecessary use of poor treatments, will often find it useful to examine the results, serially, as they become available. The ethical need to avoid extensive experimentation when treatment differences are large is characteristic of medical trials. It may arise in some types of animal experimentation, but is entirely absent from, say, agricultural field trials.

2.3. The choice of a stopping-rule

Once the way in which the treatments are to be administered has been decided – whether, for instance, each subject is to receive more than one treatment, and what administration schedule is to be used – the design of the trial is determined entirely by the stopping-rule. This lays down *in advance* the conditions under which, at any stage, the trial shall be brought to a close. What sort of stopping-rules will be suitable for medical trials; and what considerations should we have in mind in deciding which results should be associated with conclusions (a), (a)' and (b) of §1.5?

In the first place, according to the argument put forward in §1.7, stopping should be relatively early when the difference between treatment effects is sufficiently great. Secondly, it would be reasonable to insist on some control over the significance level and over the power of the procedure, as defined in §§1.5 and 1.6.

A number of different types of sequential procedure have been proposed, the most important distinction being between *open* and *closed* (or *truncated*) designs. The distinction will be clear from Fig. 2.1, which illustrates two sequential analogues of the binomial trial discussed in §§1.5 and 1.6. To use either of the charts in Fig. 2.1, a *sample path* is drawn, starting at the origin, O; for each A preference move in a 'north-easterly' direction (one unit to the right and one unit upwards); for each B preference move in a 'south-easterly' direction (one unit to the right and one downwards). Stop as soon as a boundary is hit.

In the procedure defined by the boundaries of Fig. 2.1 (a), the two outer boundaries U and L, define the results which comprise the 5 per cent. significance region. (The probability, on the null hypothesis, of reaching either of them is about 0·025.) The wedge-shaped middle boundary MM', defines the 'non-significant' region. (The dotted lines form an extension of this boundary, as explained in §3.3.) If the probability of an A preference, θ, is 0·8, the probability will be about 0·95 that the first boundary to be reached is U. Now, this procedure is 'open', in the sense that there is no limit to the distance one may travel along either of the two channels.

Fig. 2.1 (b), on the other hand, is 'closed', in the sense that the number of steps in the path (i.e. the number of preferences) is at most 40. It has very nearly the same significance level and power as the procedure of Fig. 2.1 (a) (and as the non-sequential test of §1.5).

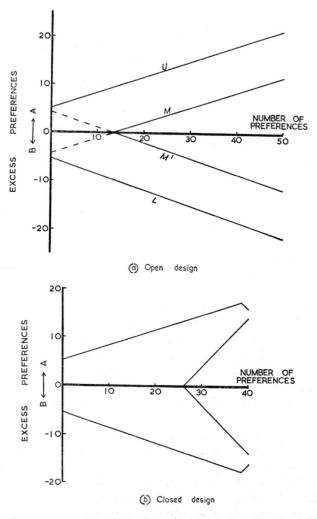

Fig. 2.1. A pair of equivalent open and closed sequential designs.

The outer boundaries of Figs. 2.1 (a) and (b) are the same straight lines. The two plans differ in the position of the middle boundary. It is clear that the open plan has the advantage of providing for earlier stoppage when the numbers of preferences are very nearly equal; MM' in the open plan would tend to be reached more quickly than the middle boundary in the closed plan. But this is counteracted by the possibility that the open plan may require rather large samples if the path wanders along the channels.

Open designs, like that of Fig. 2.1 (a) have been described previously (Armitage, 1954). A little earlier Bross (1952) described some closed designs, and I have more recently (1957) shown how to obtain a wide class of designs of this type, called *restricted procedures*. It now seems fairly clear that closed designs are the more suitable for medical trials, since the possibility that an unexpectedly long series of observations may be required is a considerable disadvantage. The general effect of using a closed rather than an open design is that the *variability* of sample size is reduced, since very small and very large samples both become less likely. However, closed designs preserve the feature, the importance of which has previously been emphasized, that the greatest reductions in sample size occur when the greatest differences between treatments are observed.

In this book, attention is devoted mainly to closed designs, although some reference is made also to open designs.

A further modification is provided by *skew designs*. If the path formed by charting the results entered the channel between M' and L in Fig. 2.1 (a) or the lower of the two pointed areas in Fig. 2.1 (b), the upper boundary could not subsequently be reached. The only conclusion that could be reached would be (a) that B is preferable to A, or (b) that no significant difference can be detected. In some trials, even though it were admitted that a difference *might* exist in either direction, it would be regarded as unethical or undesirable to prolong the investigation beyond this point. This view might well be adopted if B were a 'standard' treatment, and A were a new treatment. One might then be willing to stop the trial as soon as it was clear that the new treatment, A, was not significantly *better* than the standard treatment, B.

Skew designs will be discussed in more detail in later chapters, particularly §3.7. A point to note here is that skew designs are not incompatible with two-sided significance tests. In the type of investigation discussed in the last paragraph, more observations are required on the average when A is better than B than when B is better than A; the power curve is consequently steeper when $\theta > \frac{1}{2}$ than when $\theta < \frac{1}{2}$. Nevertheless, a verdict in favour of B may still be possible if its advantage over A is sufficiently strong.

2.4. Circumstances making sequential methods unsuitable

For some medical trials sequential methods would be unsuitable or even entirely impracticable. We mention here three of the principal difficulties.

(i) It is desirable, when applying a sequential design, that the response on which the stopping-rule is based should be available soon after treatment is started, or at any rate within a period of time which is short in comparison with the period during which subjects enter the trial. Otherwise, the number of responses available for use in the sequential analysis at any stage is considerably less than the number of treatment periods which have been started, and there is relatively little scope for economizing in the number of observations.

Sequential methods are therefore particularly suitable for trials to assess the treatment of acute conditions, or those in which rapid relief of a chronic condition is sought. Trials of long-term treatment of chronic disease, where the measurement of response can be made only after a long follow-up period, are much less amenable to sequential methods. Even in these situations, however, some sort of sequential analysis of the results available at any stage may be called for, on ethical grounds, and we shall examine the problem in more detail in Chapter 7.

A similar problem is present in many prophylactic trials for which long observations periods are required because attack rates are low.

(ii) Since the sequential analysis provides a definite instruction whether or not to stop at any stage, the response on which it is based should preferably be one of predominant importance in the assessment of the treatments. If a decision is made to stop quickly because a large difference is recorded on the chosen response, we must be prepared to forego a high degree of precision in the comparison of other responses. If death or survival is at issue, a response based on mortality will clearly be of overriding importance. In some situations there may be a number of responses of more or less equal importance, and the alternatives seem to be either to form a stopping-rule by some sort of combination of the different responses, or to carry out a non-sequential trial. The latter choice is probably the better if the condition studied is so mild that ethical considerations are unimportant.

(iii) In large-scale trials involving the co-operation of many centres, such as the trials in the chemotherapy of tuberculosis organized by the Medical Research Council, a sequential analysis may present some problems. In the first place, uncertainty about the ultimate length of the trial may cause administrative difficulties if special staff have to be employed or if a firm estimate of the total cost is required before the start of the trial. Secondly, it may be a little more troublesome to arrange for records to be sent to some central point, throughout the trial and without undue delay, than to leave the collection of records until the end. These objections are perhaps not as weighty as they at first appear, and I believe they can usually be overcome.

There are perhaps some situations in which sequential analysis *could* be applied, but where ethical considerations are so nearly negligible that a trial of predetermined size is unobjectionable. A comparison of different treatments for the common cold would perhaps be a case in point.

2.5. Pairing and randomization

In all the sequential methods for the comparison of two treatments which are described in this book, the experimental design will require that observations be made in pairs — one for each treatment. For within-subject comparisons, a natural method is to pair two successive observations on the same subject, the order of allocation to the two treatments being determined at random. For between-subject comparisons, successive subjects entered into the trial can form a pair, the allocation to the two treatments again being random.

This device is not necessary in all situations in which a sequential analysis is made on a comparative experiment. But it happens to be particularly convenient. In within-subject comparisons, any sort of statistical analysis must take account of the fact that repeated observations on the same subject form natural 'blocks' in the design, as explained in §1.4. In between-subject comparisons, the pairing of successive entrants may seem a little arbitrary. The position here is that if the response is 'all-or-none' (as, for instance, death or survival), the most suitable method of sequential analysis, to be described in Chapter 4, requires that subjects be paired. If the response is measured (Chapters 5 and 6) an analysis without pairing *can* be carried out, but it happens to be more convenient with pairs. In any case, pairing does not appreciably reduce the efficiency of the design. Little is lost, and some efficiency may be gained. For suppose there is some variability with time in the general level of the response — because of fluctuations either in the type of subject entering the trial, or in the method of assessment of response. The subjects entering the trial successively will be more alike in their response, on the average, than patients chosen randomly from the whole series, and the proposed method of pairing introduces a useful blocking system and diminishes the relevant random variation.

If there are natural subdivisions, or strata, of the population, defined perhaps by severity of disease, pairing should be carried out *within* these strata. In a trial to compare treatments for tetanus, for instance, a particular stratum may consist of young adult men, treated within 3 days of first symptoms. The first two men entered into this stratum would be allocated at random to the two treatments, and a separate random allocation applied to each subsequent pair in this stratum.

One disadvantage in pairing is that at any stage of the trial there may be some subjects left unpaired. If the design calls for no stratification, there will be at most one unpaired individual, and the loss in efficiency is negligible. With considerable stratification, there may be up to one unpaired individual in each stratum, and the loss may be more serious. For this reason care should be taken not to indulge in too much stratification unless the number of observations is likely to be very large. The number of strata should, if possible, be smaller than the smallest number of observations required by the stopping-rule.

If there are a large number of strata, a relatively high proportion of the observations may be unpaired during the initial stages of the trial. During this initial period, therefore, it may be worth carrying out a subsidiary analysis using unstratified pairs, in case a very large difference between treatments can be detected quickly.

The random allocation should be prepared before the start of the trial, and it is worth making the list for each stratum rather longer than appears to be necessary, in case the proportions of subjects falling into the different strata depart appreciably from those expected. The allocation for each pair of observations can be done by tossing a coin. Alternatively, a table of random sampling numbers can be used. If the two treatments are denoted by A and B, an *even* random digit can be taken to indicate the order AB, an *odd* digit indicating BA. Thus one random digit is required for each pair of observations.

Suppose, for instance, that in making the allocation for a particular stratum the following digits were read from part of a table of random numbers:

$$1 5 2 6 1 4 \ldots$$

The allocation would then be as follows:

$$B A \ B A \ A B \ A B \ B A \ A B \ldots$$

This system of allocation has the disadvantage that, for between-subject comparisons in which the treatments are not disguised in any way, the physician knows, for the second member of each pair, which treatment is to be used. He might occasionally be influenced (or be thought by a critic to have been influenced) by this knowledge in deciding whether or not a particular patient should enter the trial. To avoid this difficulty an allocation list can be prepared in which, within each stratum, each successive group of 4 (or 6 or 8) patients contains an equal number allocated to A and B. To achieve a balance after every 6, for instance, select a column of digits from a table of random numbers, and write down the first three numbers to occur out of the numbers 1–6. If these are, say, 4, 3 and 6, then treatment A will be allocated to the third, fourth and sixth patient in this group, and the others will receive B. The order for this group of 6 will thus be

$$B\ B\ A\ A\ B\ A.$$

If the precise system used is not divulged by the person who constructs the list, the possible bias mentioned above will probably be avoided. In the sequential analysis the first A in each balanced group is paired with the first B; the second A with the second B; and so on. Thus, in the example above three pairs will be formed by the first and third subjects; the second and fourth; and the fifth and sixth.

2.6. The comparison of more than two treatments

If more than two treatments are to be compared simultaneously the methods of allocation described in the previous section can be generalized in a fairly obvious way. Suppose there are four treatments, A, B, C and D. By analogy with simple randomized pairing, the subjects in any one strata (or the serial observations on any one patient) would be allocated randomly, in groups of four, to the different treatments. This may be arranged by writing down the digits 1–4 in the order in which they occur in random number tables, and repeating the process.

If an allocation balanced after, say, every eight subjects is required, the digits 1–8 are taken in random order, from tables of random numbers (or from tables of random permutations like Table 15.6 of Cochran and Cox (1957)). For example, the order might be

$$8\ 1\ 5\ 3\ 4\ 2\ 6\ 7.$$

Then subjects 1 and 8 are allocated to A; subjects 3 and 5 to B; 2 and 4 to C; 6 and 7 to D.

If not more than four treatments are used (and it is usually rather difficult to administer a trial with more than this number), it will probably be most informative to compare the treatments in pairs. If one treatment is shown to be significantly less effective than another it could be dropped from the trial, which would then proceed with the remaining treatments. Snell and Armitage (1957) comparing two active drugs for the suppression of cough and one placebo, found each of the active drugs to be significantly better than the placebo after the trial had run for about two-thirds of the maximum duration prescribed in advance. As it happened, only a few more observations were required to bring the third comparison – that between the two active drugs – to a close, with no significant difference demonstrated, but if this comparison had not been so nearly complete, the placebo would have been dropped. (For a fuller description of this trial, see Example 3.3.)

It should be remembered that if each treatment is to be compared with, say, two or three others, the chance that anyone will be deemed inferior to one of the others, even though they are really all equally good, is higher than it would be for a single comparison. For this reason it might be wise, when making multiple comparisons, to base the outer boundaries on rather smaller values of α than would otherwise be chosen.

CHAPTER THREE

EVALUATION BY PREFERENCES

3.1. General

In many clinical trials it is convenient to assess the relative merits of two treatments by collecting a series of qualitative preferences in favour of one or other treatment. If two treatments, A and B, are equally effective, a suitable experimental design with randomization will ensure that the observed series of preferences is a *random binomial sequence*, in which the probability of a preference in favour of A is $\frac{1}{2}$. By a 'random binomial sequence' we mean a series in which the A's and B's alternate with no systematic pattern. In situations where the preferences form a binomial sequence, we shall denote by θ the probability that a preference is an A; that is, in an indefinitely long sequence, θ would be the proportion of A preferences. The null hypothesis, then, is that $\theta = \frac{1}{2}$.

If A is really better than B, so that the null hypothesis is not true, the proportion of A preferences in the long run will be greater than $\frac{1}{2}$; and if B is preferable, the proportion of A preferences will be less than $\frac{1}{2}$. It may be, under these circumstances, that the preferences no longer form a binomial sequence with a constant value of θ. For instance, if the type of patient entering the trial changes gradually as the trial proceeds, θ may be higher (or lower) at the beginning of the trial than at the end. Nevertheless, we can consider, as one *possible* departure from the null hypothesis, a situation in which θ takes some constant value, say θ_1, greater than $\frac{1}{2}$; or (if B is the better treatment) a constant value, θ_0, less than $\frac{1}{2}$.

We could then require that our sequential procedure has a certain significance level, 2α, and has a high power of detecting a change of θ from $\frac{1}{2}$ to θ_1, or from $\frac{1}{2}$ to θ_0.

For simplicity we shall suppose that θ_0 and θ_1 are symmetrical about the value $\frac{1}{2}$; that is, $\theta_0 = 1 - \theta_1$.

3

3.2. Types of preferences

Evaluation by preferences may be suitable in a wide variety of types of trial. We may distinguish first between comparisons made within subjects, and those made between subjects. In the within-subject comparison each subject is given each treatment (possibly more than once) in a random order, and a preference is expressed by the patient or doctor on the basis of the apparent benefit derived from each treatment. In the between-subject comparison subjects are paired (as described in §2.5), and one member of each pair receives treatment A, the other subject receiving treatment B; a preference is then made by the doctor by comparing the progress of the two subjects.

The observations on which the preferences are based may vary widely in their degree of objectivity. At one extreme are subjective judgments made by the patients, as in the trial of cough suppressants (Snell and Armitage, 1957) described in §3.4. At the other extreme are observations of complete objectivity (such as death or survival), or ones in which a fairly objective measurement is made, as in the trial of hypotensive agents (Robertson and Armitage, 1959) described in §3.4. Occupying an intermediate position, perhaps, are subjective judgments made by the doctor. In this connection it should be remembered that many observations which are often thought to be fairly objective, such as X-ray assessments, have been shown sometimes to have a poor degree of reproducibility, even in repeated readings by the same observer (Fletcher and Oldham, 1959).

Qualitative preferences based on a comparison of measurements (as in the trial by Robertson and Armitage) are inefficient, in that some valuable information is lost when the actual values of the measurements are ignored. The use of preferences is valid, but not quite as efficient as the methods described in Chapter 6.

A particular case of the between-subject comparison occurs when the responses are all-or-none; for example, whether or not a patient shows a remission of symptoms in a chronic disease. This situation is sufficiently important to be considered separately, and is dealt with in Chapter 4.

3.3. Open designs

The distinction between open and closed designs has been made in §2.3. Open designs are probably less valuable in medical work than closed designs, but it will be useful to consider them briefly.

The analysis is performed graphically, on ordinary squared graph

Table 3.1. Open sequential designs for a series of preferences. (Two-sided significance level, $2\alpha = 0.05$; power $1 - \beta = 0.95$ of detecting critical values of θ.)

Critical values of θ		Coefficients in equations of boundaries			Approximate mean number of preferences required			Number of preferences required in equivalent non-sequential procedure
θ_1	$\theta_0(= 1 - \theta_1)$	a_1	a_2	b	(a) when $\theta = \frac{1}{2}$	(b) when $\theta = \theta_0$ or θ_1	(c) at max.	
0·55	0·45	36·25	29·61	0·0501	870	660	1,080	1,294
0·60	0·40	17·94	14·65	0·1007	215	160	270	319
0·65	0·35	11·75	9·60	0·1524	95	70	115	138
0·70	0·30	8·59	7·01	0·2058	51	40	63	75
0·75	0·25	6·62	5·41	0·2619	31	25	38	46
0·80	0·20	5·25	4·29	0·3219	21	17	25	30
0·85	0·15	4·19	3·42	0·3882	15	12	17	20
0·90	0·10	3·31	2·70	0·4650	10	9	11	14
0·95	0·05	2·47	2·02	0·5640	7	7	7	9

Table 3.2. Open sequential designs for a series of preferences. (Two-sided significance level, $2\alpha = 0.01$; power $1 - \beta = 0.95$ of detecting critical values of θ.)

Critical values of θ		Coefficients in equations of boundaries			Approximate mean number of preferences required			Number of preferences required in equivalent non-sequential procedure
θ_1	$\theta_0(= 1 - \theta_1)$	a_1	a_2	b	(a) when $\theta = \frac{1}{2}$	(b) when $\theta = \theta_0$ or θ_1	(c) at max.	
0·55	0·45	52·30	29·81	0·0501	928	965	1,563	1,774
0·60	0·40	25·88	14·75	0·1007	229	240	386	439
0·65	0·35	16·95	9·66	0·1524	101	106	168	191
0·70	0·30	12·39	7·06	0·2058	54	59	91	105
0·75	0·25	9·55	5·44	0·2619	33	37	56	64
0·80	0·20	7·57	4·31	0·3219	22	25	36	43
0·85	0·15	6·05	3·45	0·3882	16	18	25	29
0·90	0·10	4·78	2·72	0·4650	11	13	17	20
0·95	0·05	3·56	2·03	0·5640	7	10	11	14

paper. The entries in Table 3.1 enable the boundaries to be drawn for a series of designs having, approximately, (a) a two-sided significance level $2\alpha = 0\cdot05$, and (b) a power $1 - \beta = 0\cdot95$ of obtaining a significant result when $\theta = \theta_0$ or θ_1. Table 3.2 gives the corresponding constants for designs with $2\alpha = 0\cdot01$. The interpretation of the tabulated values is shown in Fig. 3.1. The horizontal scale measures n, the number of preferences recorded at any stage; the vertical scale measures y, the 'excess preferences', that is, the differences between the number of preferences in favour of treatment A and the number in favour of B. The results are plotted as a zig-zag line (the *sample path*) starting at O, and moving one unit diagonally upwards ('north-east') for each A preference and one unit diagonally downwards ('south-east') for each B preference.

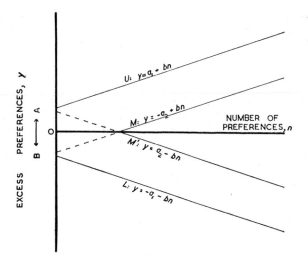

Fig. 3.1. Schematic representation of open design for a series of preferences.

The equations of the outer boundaries (indicating a significant difference between treatments) are:

$$U : y = \quad a_1 + bn$$
$$L : y = -a_1 - bn$$

The equations of the inner boundaries (which bring the trial to a close with no significant difference established) are:

$$M \ : y = -a_2 + bn$$
$$M' : y = \ \ a_2 - bn$$

The constants a_1, a_2, $-a_1$ and $-a_2$ are the intercepts of the boundaries on the y-axis; b and $-b$ represent the slopes of the lines. The dotted lines form an extension of the inner boundaries. If the sample path crosses *both* the dotted lines, the trial stops, with no significant difference established.

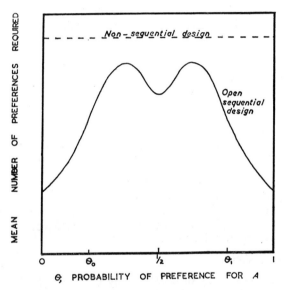

Fig. 3.2. Relationship between the average number of preferences required before a boundary is reached and the probability, θ, of an A preference, for an open sequential design and an equivalent non-sequential design.

The Tables give the mean number of preferences needed before a boundary is reached (a) when $\theta = \frac{1}{2}$ (the null hypothesis), (b) when $\theta = \theta_0$ or θ_1, and (c) in the most unfavourable circumstances, which occur when θ is about half-way between $\frac{1}{2}$ and θ_0, or between $\frac{1}{2}$ and θ_1 (when the sample path tends to go in the direction of one of the channels between the parallel boundaries). The sample-size of a non-sequential procedure with the same properties is also shown; a non-sequential sample of this number of preferences would have the same significance level, 2α, and the same power, $1 - \beta$, of detecting a value of θ equal to θ_0 or θ_1. The mean number of preferences clearly varies appreciably with the true value of θ, and the relationship is in general similar to that shown in Fig. 3.2. Even in the least favourable situation, the sequential design is more economical than the non-sequential procedure. But we must emphasize that these results refer to the *average* number of preferences required, over a series of imaginary repetitions of the trial. In an individual instance we may need less than the average, or more, and it is clear from the nature of the boundaries that we *may* need very many more — if the path wanders along either channel. The variability of sample size about its average is, in fact, very considerable, and it is mainly in order to reduce this variability that closed schemes have been introduced.

Example 3.1

Sainsbury and Lucas (1959) reported a trial to assess the efficacy of pro-chlorperazine in reducing tension and anxiety in psychoneurotic patients. Each patient received prochlorperazine for a period of a week, and an indistinguishable placebo for a week. The order was determined randomly and was unknown to the doctor. The response to treatment during each week was scored on a five-point scale, and at the end of the two weeks a preference was recorded if the patient's score on one treatment was greater than his score on the other treatment. When the scores were equal no preference was recorded.

The authors used the open design with $2\alpha = 0 \cdot 05$, $1 - \beta = 0 \cdot 95$, $\theta_1 = 0 \cdot 8$. After 14 preferences had been recorded one of the inner boundaries was reached and the trial stopped, no significant difference between the treatments having been discovered. Six patients provided no preference. A total of 20 patients therefore entered the trial.

3.4. Closed designs

To avoid the possibility of exceptionally large sample sizes the open designs described in the last section can be 'truncated', by allowing the outer and inner boundaries to meet at some distance up the channels. But unless the truncation is performed a long way up the channels the designs no longer provide the required risks α and β. Truncation at sample sizes large enough to preserve approximately the required risks diminishes slightly, but does not remove, the difficulty.

Bross's designs

Bross (1952) was the first to suggest the use of specially constructed closed designs, as distinct from arbitrarily truncated open designs, and his paper contains details of two such schemes. The boundaries are shown in Figs. 3.3 and 3.4. For the sake of uniformity we use here the same form of graphical presentation as is used elsewhere in this chapter, although Bross uses a different form of diagram in which the two

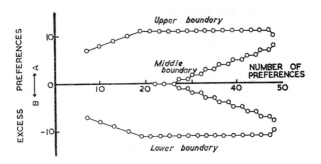

Fig. 3.3. Bross's plan *A*.

co-ordinate axes represent the numbers of each type of preference. The reader may prefer to use Bross's form of chart, and in any case he will find it profitable to compare the two pairs of diagrams. Bross describes the use of his designs in terms of the problem of comparing two success-rates, which we shall consider in Chapter 4, but they are applicable for any type of preferences. Owing to the discontinuous nature of the steps taken by the sample path, there is only a certain number of points at which the boundaries can be crossed. These boundary points are shown by circles in Figs. 3.3 and 3.4, and their co-ordinates are given in Table 3.3.

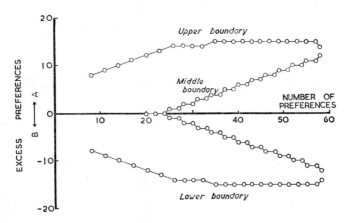

Fig. 3.4. Bross's plan *B*.

Table 3.3. Specification of boundary points for Bross's closed sequential designs.

| | Plan A | | | Plan B | |
| | Excess preferences y | | | | y | |
Number of preferences n	Upper bound.	Lower bound.	n	Upper bound.	Lower bound.
7	7	−7	8	8	−8
10	8	−8	11	9	−9
13	9	−9	14	10	−10
16	10	−10	17	11	−11
19	11	−11	20	12	−12
21	11	−11	23	13	−13
23	11	−11	26	14	−14
25	11	−11	28	14	−14
27	11	−11	30	14	−14
29	11	−11	32	14	−14
31	11	−11	35	15	−15
33	11	−11	37	15	−15
35	11	−11	39	15	−15
37	11	−11	41	15	−15
39	11	−11	43	15	−15
41	11	−11	45	15	−15
43	11	−11	47	15	−15
45	11	−11	49	15	−15
47	11	−11	51	15	−15
48	10	−10	53	15	−15
			55	15	−15
			57	15	−15
			58	14	−14

Plan A — Middle boundary

n	Upper	Lower
48	8	−8
47	7	−7
45	7	−7
44	6	−6
42	6	−6
41	5	−5
39	5	−5
38	4	−4
36	4	−4
35	3	−3
33	3	−3
32	2	−2
30	2	−2
29	1	−1
27	1	−1
26	0	
24	0	
22	0	

Plan B — Middle boundary

n	Upper	Lower
58	12	−12
57	11	−11
55	11	−11
54	10	−10
52	10	−10
51	9	−9
49	9	−9
48	8	−8
46	8	−8
45	7	−7
43	7	−7
42	6	−6
40	6	−6
39	5	−5
37	5	−5
36	4	−4
34	4	−4
33	3	−3
31	3	−3
30	2	−2
28	2	−2
27	1	−1
25	1	−1
24	0	
22	0	
20	0	

Table 3.4. Some properties of Bross's closed designs.

		Plan *A*	Plan *B*
Probability, $2a$, of reaching outer boundaries on null hypothesis that $\theta = \frac{1}{2}$		0·215	0·098
Probability of reaching upper boundary when	$\theta = 0·6$	0·500	0·371
	$\theta = 0·7$	0·905	0·860

Some of the properties of Bross's designs are given in his paper, and are reproduced in Table 3.4.

Example 3.2

An example of the use of Bross's plan *B* is provided by a double-blind trial reported by Newton and Tanner (1956), to compare the effectiveness of *N*-acetyl-para-aminophenol (N.A.P.A.P.) and tab. codein co. as analgesics. Patients needing relief of pain were given one of the two types of tablet for a

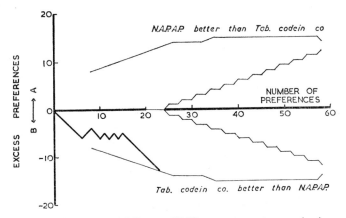

Fig. 3.5. Trial of Newton and Tanner (1956) to compare two analgesics, using Bross's plan *B*. Sample path shown by thick line.

period of a week, and the other treatment was used for the following week, the order of administration being chosen randomly. The whole procedure was then repeated for a further two-weekly period, the order of administration again being randomized. At the end of each two-weekly period patients were asked to state a preference between the two treatments they had received. In the main analysis only those patients who gave two consistent preferences were considered. The series of preferences is plotted in Fig. 3.5, from which it will be seen that N.A.P.A.P. was shown to be inferior to tab. codein co. after 23 preferences (of which 18 favoured tab. codein co. and 5 favoured N.A.P.A.P.). At this stage 42 patients had been treated. An interesting feature of this experimental scheme is that it provides evidence on the extent to which patients gave consistent preferences in one or other direction. The results suggest that patients differ in their degree of preference for tab. codein co., and that quite possibly a minority of patients prefer N.A.P.A.P. For further discussion see Newton and Tanner's paper, and also a note by Armitage and Healy (1957).

Some other trials of analgesics, using Bross's plan B, are reported by Thomson (1958).

Restricted designs

A class of sequential designs, called *restricted procedures*, was introduced by Armitage (1957). These designs are similar to those of Bross, but provide a much wider choice. The shape of the boundaries is

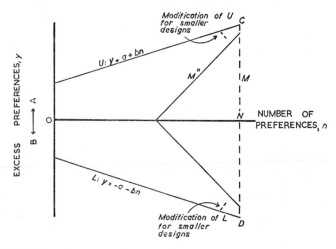

Fig. 3.6. Schematic representation of restricted design. In some of the smaller designs (cf. Fig. 2.1 (b)) U and L have been slightly curtailed as indicated by the broken line, to bring a close to the nominal value.

illustrated by Fig. 3.6. The equations of the upper and lower boundaries are, respectively,

$$U : y = a + bn$$

and

$$L : y = -a - bn.$$

The maximum number of preferences required is N. The points on the upper and lower boundaries, when $n = N$, are denoted by C and D, respectively. The middle boundary can take the form of a straight line (M) at $n = N$; alternatively a modified boundary, M'', can be drawn in the shape of a wedge at an angle of $45°$ to the horizontal, from the extreme points on M (the highest accessible point below C and the lowest accessible point above D). The reason why the middle boundary

Table 3.5. Restricted sequential designs for a series of preferences. (Two-sided significance level, $2\alpha = 0.05$; power $1 - \beta = 0.95$ of detecting critical values of θ.)

Critical values of θ		Coefficients in equations of boundaries		Maximum number of preferences required	Exact values of probabilities of reaching outer boundaries	
θ_1	$\theta_0(= 1 - \theta_1)$	a	b	N	2α	$1 - \beta$
0·55	0·45	36·25	0·0501	1,778	Not calculated	
0·60	0·40	17·94	0·1007	439		
0·65	0·35	11·75	0·1524	191		
0·70	0·30	8·59	0·2058	104		
0·75	0·25	See Table 3.7 for boundary points		62	0·047	0·965
0·80	0·20			40	0·047	0·964
0·85	0·15			27	0·047	0·967
0·90	0·10			19	0·041	0·970
0·95	0·05			13	0·048	0·979

Table 3.6. Restricted sequential designs for a series of preferences. (Two-sided significance level, $2\alpha = 0.01$; power $1 - \beta = 0.95$ of detecting critical values of θ.)

Critical values of θ		Coefficients in equations of boundaries		Maximum number of preferences required	Exact values of probabilities of reaching outer boundaries	
θ_1	$\theta_0(= 1 - \theta_1)$	a	b	N	2α	$1 - \beta$
0·55	0·45	52·30	0·0501	2,290	Not calculated	
0·60	0·40	25·88	0·1007	565		
0·65	0·35	16·95	0·1524	244		
0·70	0·30	12·39	0·2058	132		
0·75	0·25	9·55	0·2619	80		
0·80	0·20	See Table 3.8 for boundary points		49	0·009	0·955
0·85	0·15			33	0·010	0·955
0·90	0·10			22	0·010	0·944
0·95	0·05			16	0·008	0·961

may take this modified form is that any sample path which reaches M'' could not possibly cross either the upper or the lower boundaries even if the trial continued until N preferences had been recorded (since the sample path cannot move at a steeper angle than 45°, upwards or downwards).

Some theoretical results enable one to obtain reasonable approximations to a, b and N, for designs having (a) a particular two-sided significance level, 2α, and (b) a particular power, $1 - \beta$, of obtaining a significant result (i.e. hitting either the upper or the lower boundary) when $\theta = \theta_0$ or θ_1. The first few entries in Tables 3.5 and 3.6 give the values of these constants for $2\alpha = 0\cdot05$ and $0\cdot01$, respectively, and $1 - \beta = 0\cdot95$ in each case. It will be noted that a and b are the same as the corresponding values of a_1 and b in Tables 3.1 and 3.2. Thus, the outer boundaries of the corresponding open and closed designs coincide. Fig. 2.1 shows a pair of equivalent designs. The effect of using a restricted procedure rather than the corresponding open design is clearly to reduce the possibility that a very large number of observations will be needed, and also to increase the minimum number of observations when the preferences occur with equal frequency.

The lower entries in Tables 3.5 and 3.6 refer to smaller designs (i.e. with smaller values of N), and for these it has been possible to work out the exact probabilities of reaching the various boundary points (see Appendix A.4). Slight amendments have been made to the boundaries obtained by the theoretical approximation (as given in Table 5 of Armitage, 1957) in order to make α slightly less than, but very close to, the required value. The exact values of 2α and $1 - \beta$ are shown in the Tables; the values of $1 - \beta$ are usually rather greater than the nominal value of $0\cdot95$.

The exact specifications for the smaller designs are given in Tables 3.7 and 3.8. These give details of the boundary points, and also the cumulative probabilities (on the null hypothesis) of reaching the various points on the outer boundaries.

Example 3.3

Snell and Armitage (1957) used the design with $2\alpha = 0\cdot05$, $1 - \beta = 0\cdot05$, $\theta_1 = 0\cdot85$, $N = 27$* in a trial of cough suppressants. There were three treatments, heroin (diamorphine), 'lipect' (pholcodine) and a placebo, and these were administered in a random order to patients with chronic cough. Each treatment was prepared in the form of a linctus, and each patient received a particular linctus on two successive evenings, and at the end of six

---

* Actually the design was closed at $N = 30$, this being the theoretical approximation corresponding to the more exact value $N = 27$.

Table 3.7. Restricted designs for a series of preferences. Exact specification of boundary points for the smaller restricted designs (Two-sided significance level, $2\alpha = 0.05$; power $1 - \beta = 0.95$ of detecting critical values of θ.)

$\theta_1 = 0.75$

Number of prefs. n	Excess preferences y		Cumulative prob. of given result or more extreme, P
	Upper bound U	Lower bound L	
9	9	−9	0.004
12	10	−10	0.008
15	11	−11	0.012
18	12	−12	0.015
20	12	−13	0.020
23	13	−14	0.023
26	14	−14	0.026
28	14	−15	0.029
31	15	−15	0.031
34	16	−16	0.033
37	17	−17	0.034
39	17	−17	0.036
42	18	−18	0.037
45	19	−19	0.038
47	19	−19	0.039
50	20	−20	0.039
53	21	−21	0.040
56	22	−22	0.040
58	22	−22	0.041
60	22	−22	0.042
61	21	−21	0.044
62	20	−20	0.047

Modified middle boundary M''; straight lines joining:
$$\left\{ \begin{array}{cc} n & y \\ (44, & 0) \\ \text{to } (62, & 18) \end{array} \right. \quad \text{and} \quad \left\{ \begin{array}{cc} (44, & 0) \\ \text{to } (62, & -18) \end{array} \right.$$

$\theta_1 = 0.80$

n	U	L (y)	P
8	8	−8	0.008
11	9	−9	0.016
14	10	−10	0.022
17	11	−11	0.027
20	12	−12	0.031
23	13	−13	0.033
26	13	−14	0.035
29	14	−15	0.037
32	15	−16	0.038
35	16	−17	0.039
38	17	−17	0.040
39	17	−17	0.042
40	16	−16	0.047

$$M'' \left\{ \begin{array}{cc} n & y \\ (26, & 0) \\ \text{to } (40, & 14) \end{array} \right. \quad \text{and} \quad \left\{ \begin{array}{cc} (26, & 0) \\ \text{to } (40, & -14) \end{array} \right.$$

$\theta_1 = 0.85$

n	U	L (y)	P
7	7	−7	0.016
11	9	−9	0.022
14	10	−10	0.028
17	11	−11	0.033
20	12	−12	0.037
24	14	−14	0.038
26	14	−14	0.041
27	13	−13	0.047

$$M'' \left\{ \begin{array}{cc} n & y \\ (16, & 0) \\ \text{to } (27, & 11) \end{array} \right. \quad \text{and} \quad \left\{ \begin{array}{cc} (16, & 0) \\ \text{to } (27, & -11) \end{array} \right.$$

$\theta_1 = 0.90$

n	U	L (y)	P
7	7	−7	0.016
10	8	−8	0.029
14	10	−10	0.034
18	12	−12	0.037
19	11	−11	0.041

$$M'' \left\{ \begin{array}{cc} n & y \\ (10, & 0) \\ \text{to } (19, & 9) \end{array} \right. \quad \text{and} \quad \left\{ \begin{array}{cc} (10, & 0) \\ \text{to } (19, & -9) \end{array} \right.$$

$\theta_1 = 0.95$

n	U	L (y)	P
6	6	−6	0.032
11	9	−9	0.038
13	9	−9	0.048

$$M'' \left\{ \begin{array}{cc} n & y \\ (6, & 0) \\ \text{to } (13, & 7) \end{array} \right. \quad \text{and} \quad \left\{ \begin{array}{cc} (6, & 0) \\ \text{to } (13, & -7) \end{array} \right.$$

Table 3.8. Restricted designs for a series of preferences. Exact specification of boundary points for the restricted designs. (Two-sided significance level, $2\alpha = 0\cdot01$; power $1 - \beta = 0\cdot95$ of detecting critical values of θ.)

$\theta_1 = 0\cdot80$

Number of prefs. n	Excess preferences y		Cumulative prob. of given result or more extreme, P
	Upper bound. U	Lower bound. L	
12	12	−12	0·0005
15	13	−13	0·0012
18	14	−14	0·0020
21	15	−15	0·0027
23	15	−15	0·0040
26	16	−16	0·0049
29	17	−17	0·0056
32	18	−18	0·0062
35	19	−19	0·0066
38	20	−20	0·0070
41	21	−21	0·0073
44	22	−22	0·0075
47	23	−23	0·0077
48	22	−22	0·0082
49	21	−21	0·0095

Modified middle boundary M'; straight lines joining

$$
M' \quad
\begin{cases}
n & y \\
(30, & 0) \\
\text{to } (49, & 19)
\end{cases}
\quad \text{and} \quad
\begin{cases}
(30, & 0) \\
\text{to } (49, & -19)
\end{cases}
$$

$\theta_1 = 0\cdot85$

n	U	L	P
10	10	−10	0·0020
14	12	−12	0·0032
17	13	−13	0·0045
20	14	−14	0·0056
23	15	−15	0·0066
27	17	−17	0·0071
30	18	−18	0·0074
32	18	−18	0·0081
33	17	−17	0·0099

$$
M'' \quad
\begin{cases}
n & y \\
(18, & 0) \\
\text{to } (33, & 15)
\end{cases}
\quad \text{and} \quad
\begin{cases}
(18, & 0) \\
\text{to } (33, & -15)
\end{cases}
$$

$\theta_1 = 0\cdot90$

n	U	L	P
9	9	−9	0·0039
13	11	−11	0·0061
17	13	−13	0·0072
21	15	−15	0·0077
22	14	−14	0·0099

$$
M'' \quad
\begin{cases}
n & y \\
(10, & 0) \\
\text{to } (22, & 12)
\end{cases}
\quad \text{and} \quad
\begin{cases}
(10, & 0) \\
\text{to } (22, & -12)
\end{cases}
$$

$\theta_1 = 0\cdot95$

n	U	L	P
9	9	−9	0·0039
13	11	−11	0·0061
16	12	−12	0·0083

$$
M'' \quad
\begin{cases}
n & y \\
(6, & 0) \\
\text{to } (16, & 10)
\end{cases}
\quad \text{and} \quad
\begin{cases}
(6, & 0) \\
\text{to } (16, & -10)
\end{cases}
$$

days (having received all three treatments) he was asked to rank them in order of preference. Some patients were unable to state a preference between some or all of the treatments, but a separate chart was used for each pair of treatments, and all available preferences were plotted sequentially. The total time span of the trial was fixed by other commitments. The rate at which preferences were becoming available was estimated from the first part of the trial, and this enabled a reasonable guess to be made of the total number of preferences which would be available for each comparison, in the maximum allowable time. These considerations led to the choice of the restricted design with $N = 27$. The completed charts are shown in Fig. 3.7. The conclusion is that heroin and 'lipect' were both preferable to the placebo, but no distinction could be made between the two active drugs. The boundaries were reached at $n = 17$, 17 and 20.

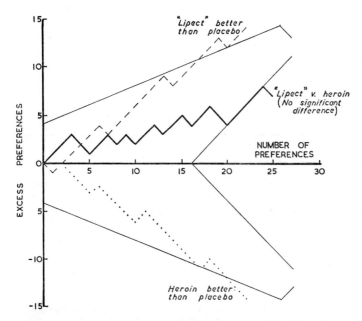

Fig. 3.7. Trial of Snell and Armitage (1957) to compare 'lipect', heroin and a placebo, as cough suppressants, using a restricted design, with $2\alpha = 0.05$, $1 - \beta = 0.95$, $\theta_1 = 0.85$, $N = 27$.

Example 3.4

Robertson and Armitage (1959) report a trial to compare two hypotensive agents, phenactropinium chloride and trimetaphan. The comparison was made *between* subjects, by comparing the times required, in pairs of subjects, for the systolic blood pressure to recover to a level of 100 mm. Hg, after it had been lowered during operation by application of one of the two drugs. We shall consider in Chapter 6 a possible sequential analysis of these data which uses the actual measurements, but at present we follow the authors in forming qualitative preferences by noting which of the two recovery times in each pair was the shorter.

The authors used the restricted design with $2\alpha = 0 \cdot 05$, $1 - \beta = 0 \cdot 05$, $\theta_1 = 0 \cdot 75$, $N = 62$. Since the drugs were used in a wide variety of operative conditions, results flowed in fairly quickly, and it was felt worthwhile to use a rather large design in order to attain a greater power. The results are shown in Fig. 3.8. The path reached the middle boundary at the 49th preference, after which one more pair of patients was treated. Only three pairs failed to provide a preference (by having equal recovery times). In all, then, 53 pairs of

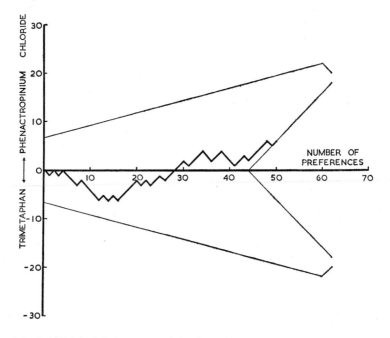

Fig. 3.8. Trial of Robertson and Armitage (1959) to compare two hypotensive agents, using a restricted design with $2\alpha = 0 \cdot 05$, $1 - \beta = 0 \cdot 95$, $\theta_1 = 0 \cdot 75$, $N = 62$.

patients were needed for the trial. An interesting point is that the first 12 preferences showed a marked preponderance for trimetaphan, which, in the whole trial, was slightly less effective than phenactropinium. If the results had not been subjected to a sequential analysis the trial might have been stopped at this early stage, and the conclusion drawn that trimetaphan was the better treatment.

For another trial using a restricted design for between-subject comparisons, see Flavell Matts (1960).

3.5. Exact significance level

It has been explained in §1.5 that in non-sequential significance tests a common procedure is to calculate the probability, on the null hypothesis, of obtaining the observed result or one showing a greater departure from that expected. This cumulative probability, P, may be regarded as the exact significance level at which the observed result is just significant.

In a sequential procedure of the types described in §§3.3 and 3.4, one possible approach is to regard a path which reaches a particular point on either of the outer boundaries as less extreme than one which reaches the same boundary at an earlier stage, since for the latter path the proportions of preferences will depart further from the expected 50 : 50 ratio. As a measure of the extent to which the null hypothesis is contradicted, then, we may calculate the cumulative probability, P, of reaching the observed point on an outer boundary or an earlier point. The values of P, for boundary points in the restricted procedures for which exact results are available, are given in Tables 3.7 and 3.8.

3.6. Confidence limits for θ

The exact specification of confidence limits, for use in sequential procedures, is a difficult problem. Some investigations by Armitage (1958) suggest that a reasonable approximation is provided by the usual methods used in non-sequential investigations. The approximation is probably better for closed than for open designs. For restricted procedures the approximation is likely to be particularly reliable for paths ending on the middle boundary.

Suppose that, at the boundary point, n preferences have been recorded, of which r are in favour of A, and $n - r$ in favour of B. Let $r/n = p$, and $q = 1 - p$. Then, if n is fairly large (say 30 or more), and if p is not too near 0 or 1, approximate 95 per cent. confidence limits for θ are given by

$$p \pm 2\sqrt{(pq/n)}.$$

If either r or $n - r$ are rather small (say 10 or less), reference may be made to the tables of Mainland *et al.* (1956). Both the approximate and the more exact results are based on non-sequential theory. For points on, say, the upper boundary of a restricted procedure, the confidence limits are both a little too high; that is, rather better values are obtained by moving the limits a little nearer $\frac{1}{2}$. Unfortunately, no simple rule for this adjustment can yet be given.

4

If the sample path reaches the middle boundary after a relatively large number of observations (for example, some way along one of the pointed areas in a restricted design), the confidence limits for θ may exclude the value $\frac{1}{2}$. There will then be a contradiction between the verdict of the sequential procedure (that the difference between A and B is non-significant), and that of the confidence limits. In such circumstances the sequential result should be preferred.

3.7. Skew designs

Skew designs were discussed briefly in §2.3. In certain trials one may be satisfied to stop as soon as it is clear that a particular one of the two outer boundaries becomes inaccessible. We shall suppose that the trial is designed primarily to detect a superiority of A over B (typically A

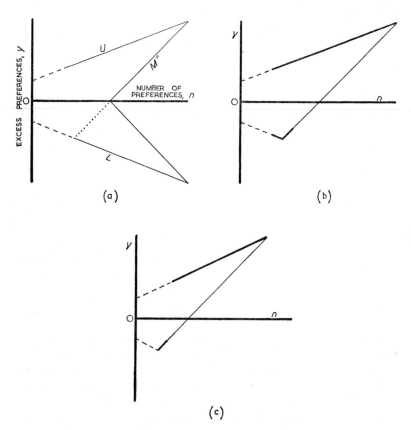

Fig. 3.9. The method of forming skew restricted designs.

would be a new treatment and B a standard treatment). The trial will stop as soon as it is clear that U cannot be reached.

The appropriate open design is formed by one pair of parallel lines, U and M.

Skew restricted designs are formed as shown in Fig. 3.9 (a), by continuing the upper arm of M'' downwards. If it crosses the accessible part of L the first portion of L may be included as part of the new boundary, as in Fig. 3.9 (b). With some of the smaller designs the continuation of the upper arm of M'' may cross the inaccessible part of L (as in Fig. 3.9 (c)); L should then be ignored entirely.

Example 3.5

In a trial of anticoagulants in the treatment of cerebral infarction, Marshall and Shaw (1960) used a restricted design with $2a = 0 \cdot 05$, $1 - \beta = 0 \cdot 95$, $\theta_1 = 0 \cdot 90$, $N = 19$. The preferences here were 'untied' pairs of patients differing in their survival experience 6 weeks after start of treatment. (This method of assessment is explained in Chapter 4, but the example is described here as it illustrates the points discussed above.) When 8 preferences had been obtained, 3 were for anticoagulants and 5 for the control treatment without anticoagulants. The path had then entered the pointed area from which the outer boundary favouring anticoagulants was inaccessible. It was regarded as unethical to continue the investigation merely to see whether anticoagulant treatment could be shown to be *worse* than the standard treatment.

Skew designs are not incompatible with two-sided significance tests. Even if, as in the example above, the main question is whether A is better than B, it will still be useful to take note of a striking preponderance of preferences for B over those for A. A small number of the most extreme boundary points on the lower and middle boundaries, having a probability of not more than a when the null hypothesis is true, may be regarded as forming a significance region. These are shown by the short sections of heavy line in Fig. 3.9 (b) and (c).

The skew versions of the designs listed in Tables 3.7 and 3.8 are tabulated in Tables 3.9 and 3.10.

A skew design has the same power as the corresponding symmetrical design when $\theta > \frac{1}{2}$ (A being superior to B), but has much lower power than $\theta < \frac{1}{2}$. This feature is illustrated in Fig. 3.10, for the restricted designs with $2a = 0 \cdot 05$, $1 - \beta = 0 \cdot 95$, $\theta_1 = 0 \cdot 8$, $N = 40$. The symmetrical design achieves higher power than the skew design for $\theta < \frac{1}{2}$ because it requires on the average more observations. Fig. 3.11 shows the mean number of preferences required by both the skew and symmetrical procedures for various values of θ.

Tables 3.9. Skew restricted designs for a series of preferences. Exact specification of boundary points for the smaller designs. (Two-sided significance level, $2a = 0·05$; power $1 − \beta = 0·95$ of detecting critical values of θ.)

	$\theta_1 = 0·75$		$\theta_1 = 0·80$		$\theta_1 = 0·85$		$\theta_1 = 0·90$		$\theta_1 = 0·95$	
	Number of prefs. n	Excess prefs. y	n	y	n	y	n	y	n	y
Upper boundary	As in Table 3.7		As in Table 3.7		As in Table 3.7		As in Table 3.7		As in Table 3.7	
Middle boundary Straight line joining	(62,	18)	(40,	14)	(27,	11)	(19,	9)	(13,	7)
to	(32,	−12)	(17,	−9)	(10,	−6)	(5,	−5)	(3,	−3)
Lower boundary	9	−9	8	−8	7	−7	None		None	
	12	−10	11	−9	9	−7				
	15	−11	14	−10						
	18	−12	16	−10						
	20	−12								
	23	−13								
	26	−14								
	28	−14								
	30	−14								
	31	−13								

Table 3.10. Skew restricted designs for a series of preferences. Exact specification of boundary points for the smaller designs. (Two-sided significance level, $2\alpha = 0.05$; power $1 - \beta$ of detecting critical values of θ.)

	$\theta_1 = 0.80$		$\theta_1 = 0.85$		$\theta_1 = 0.90$		$\theta_1 = 0.95$	
	Number of prefs. n	Excess prefs. y	n	y	n	y	n	y
Upper boundary	As in Table 3.8		As in Table 3.8		As in Table 3.8		As in Table 3.8	
Middle boundary Straight line joining	(49,	19)	(33,	15)	(22,	12)	(16,	10)
to	(19,	−11)	(10,	−8)	(5,	−5)	(3,	−3)
Lower boundary	12	−12	9	−9	None		None	
	15	−13						
	17	−13						
	18	−12						

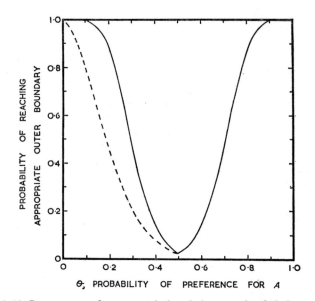

Fig. 3.10. Power curves for symmetrical and skew restricted designs with $2a = 0.05$, $1 - \beta = 0.95$, $\theta_1 = 0.8$, $N = 40$.
———— symmetrical design; – – – – – skew design. θ is probability of a preference for treatment A.

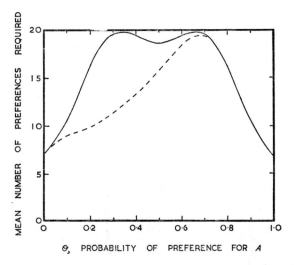

Fig. 3.11. Mean number of preferences required by symmetrical and skew restricted designs with $2a = 0.05$, $1 - \beta = 0.95$, $\theta_1 = 0.8$, $N = 40$.
———— symmetrical design; – – – – skew design. θ is the probability of a preference for treatment A.

3.8. The choice of a design

In choosing a particular design for use in a sequential trial, the same considerations apply as in any statistical investigation. The desire to improve the sensitivity (i.e. the power to detect real effects if they are present) must be balanced against the desire to economize in time and expense. The point has already been made in §1.6.

For restricted sequential trials involving preferences, Tables 3.5–3.10 enable one to compare the power of, and the maximum number of preferences required by, various alternative designs. It will be difficult to make a rational choice unless one has some idea of the rate at which preferences will become available, so that some estimate can be made of the maximum duration of the trial. There may be some reliable information as to the rate at which patients will enter the trial, but perhaps less reliable information about the proportion of possible comparisons which will yield usable preferences. If the organizers of the trial wish to estimate the rate of obtaining preferences, but feel unable to make any intelligent guess, the best plan is probably to start the trial, without any rigid boundaries, and to draw these in only when the rate of preferences can be assessed from the data.

CHAPTER FOUR

COMPARISON OF TWO PROPORTIONS

4.1. Introduction

One of the most common methods of assessing the relative efficacy of two therapeutic procedures is to form two groups of patients by random allocation in the usual way, treat one group by each therapy, and compare the proportions of patients in the two groups who show some particular favourable response (which in general we may call a *success*). The usual non-sequential technique for analysing this type of data is the χ^2 test for a 2×2 table, or the equivalent method of comparing the difference between the proportions of successes in the two groups with the standard error of this difference.

In some instances the observations in the two groups may follow some natural system of pairing. For example, in a trial in which treatments are compared within patients each patient may receive treatments A and B on successive occasions, in a random order. It is still relevant to compare the proportions of successes in the two groups, but the method of analysis must take account of the natural pairing of the observations (McNemar, 1949; Cochran, 1950). The method of analysis described by McNemar and Cochran is, in fact, to compare the number of patients who succeed on A but not on B, with the number of those who succeed on B but not on A. Those who succeed on both treatments, or fail on both, are ignored. This is essentially the device adopted in the sequential analysis described in the next section. It can be used either when the observations are naturally paired, as in the type of data just discussed, or for series like those discussed in the last paragraph in which there is no natural pairing.

We consider first the simple between-subject comparison, with random allocation of subjects to two treatment groups and no natural pairing of observations. We assume that some well-defined response criterion has been chosen, so that each patient can be classified as either a 'success' or a 'failure'.

As patients enter the trial they are formed into pairs, one treated with
A and the other with B. Methods of allocation have been discussed in
§2.5. The results for each pair will fall into one of the following categories (S denoting success, F failure):

	Patient treated with A	B	Preference for
(a)	S	S	$-\Big\}$ Tied pairs.
(b)	F	F	$-$
(c)	S	F	$A\Big\}$ Untied pairs.
(d)	F	S	B

Pairs of types (a) and (b) may be called *tied pairs*, because the comparison between treatments results in a tie. Those of types (c) and
(d) may similarly be called *untied pairs*. The untied pairs result in a
preference for one or other treatment: type (c) a preference for A, and
type (d) a preference for B. If now we record the results sequentially
we shall have a series of preferences for A or B punctuated by a number
of tied pairs yielding no preference. This is precisely the sort of series
already discussed in Chapter 3, and all the sequential designs described
there apply equally well to the present situation. There are in addition,
however, some special considerations which will be explained in the
next section.

4.2. The derived series of preferences

Suppose that the probability of a success with treatment A is π_1; that is,
the series of patients treated with A can be regarded as a random binomial sequence (see §3.1) in which the 'long-run' proportion of
successes is π_1. Similarly, suppose the probability of a success with B
is π_2.

Then, on the assumption that pairing is random we can write down
the probabilities of the four types of pair:

	Type	A	B	Preference	Probability
Tied	(a)	S	S	$-$	$\pi_1 \pi_2$
	(b)	F	F	$-$	$(1 - \pi_1)(1 - \pi_2)$
Untied	(c)	S	F	A	$\pi_1(1 - \pi_2)$
	(d)	F	S	B	$(1 - \pi_1)\pi_2$

Table 4.1. Values of ϕ and θ for various combinations of π_1 and π_2 (ϕ shown in ordinary type, θ in bold type).

π_1 → π_2 ↓	0·05	0·10	0·15	0·20	0·25	0·30	0·35	0·40	0·45	0·50	0·55	0·60	0·65	0·70	0·75	0·80	0·85	0·90	0·95
0·05	0·095	0·140	0·185	0·230	0·275	0·320	0·365	0·410	0·455	0·500	0·545	0·590	0·635	0·680	0·725	0·770	0·815	0·860	0·905
	0·500	**0·679**	**0·770**	**0·826**	**0·864**	**0·891**	**0·911**	**0·927**	**0·940**	**0·950**	**0·959**	**0·966**	**0·972**	**0·978**	**0·983**	**0·987**	**0·991**	**0·994**	**0·997**
0·10	0·140	0·180	0·220	0·260	0·300	0·340	0·380	0·420	0·460	0·500	0·540	0·580	0·620	0·660	0·700	0·740	0·780	0·820	0·860
	0·321	**0·500**	**0·614**	**0·692**	**0·750**	**0·794**	**0·829**	**0·857**	**0·880**	**0·900**	**0·917**	**0·931**	**0·944**	**0·954**	**0·964**	**0·973**	**0·981**	**0·988**	**0·994**
0·15	0·185	0·220	0·255	0·290	0·325	0·360	0·395	0·430	0·465	0·500	0·535	0·570	0·605	0·640	0·675	0·710	0·745	0·780	0·815
	0·230	**0·386**	**0·500**	**0·586**	**0·654**	**0·708**	**0·753**	**0·791**	**0·823**	**0·850**	**0·874**	**0·895**	**0·913**	**0·930**	**0·944**	**0·958**	**0·970**	**0·981**	**0·991**
0·20	0·230	0·260	0·290	0·320	0·350	0·380	0·410	0·440	0·470	0·500	0·530	0·560	0·590	0·620	0·650	0·680	0·710	0·740	0·770
	0·174	**0·308**	**0·414**	**0·500**	**0·571**	**0·632**	**0·683**	**0·727**	**0·766**	**0·800**	**0·830**	**0·857**	**0·881**	**0·903**	**0·923**	**0·941**	**0·958**	**0·973**	**0·987**
0·25	0·275	0·300	0·325	0·350	0·375	0·400	0·425	0·450	0·475	0·500	0·525	0·550	0·575	0·600	0·625	0·650	0·675	0·700	0·725
	0·136	**0·250**	**0·346**	**0·429**	**0·500**	**0·562**	**0·618**	**0·667**	**0·710**	**0·750**	**0·786**	**0·818**	**0·848**	**0·875**	**0·900**	**0·923**	**0·944**	**0·964**	**0·983**
0·30	0·320	0·340	0·360	0·380	0·400	0·420	0·440	0·460	0·480	0·500	0·520	0·540	0·560	0·580	0·600	0·620	0·640	0·660	0·680
	0·109	**0·206**	**0·292**	**0·368**	**0·438**	**0·500**	**0·557**	**0·609**	**0·656**	**0·700**	**0·740**	**0·778**	**0·812**	**0·845**	**0·875**	**0·903**	**0·930**	**0·954**	**0·978**
0·35	0·365	0·380	0·395	0·410	0·425	0·440	0·455	0·470	0·485	0·500	0·515	0·530	0·545	0·560	0·575	0·590	0·605	0·620	0·635
	0·089	**0·171**	**0·247**	**0·317**	**0·382**	**0·443**	**0·500**	**0·553**	**0·603**	**0·650**	**0·694**	**0·736**	**0·775**	**0·812**	**0·848**	**0·881**	**0·913**	**0·944**	**0·972**
0·40	0·410	0·420	0·430	0·440	0·450	0·460	0·470	0·480	0·490	0·500	0·510	0·520	0·530	0·540	0·550	0·560	0·570	0·580	0·590
	0·073	**0·143**	**0·209**	**0·273**	**0·333**	**0·391**	**0·447**	**0·500**	**0·551**	**0·600**	**0·647**	**0·692**	**0·736**	**0·778**	**0·818**	**0·857**	**0·895**	**0·931**	**0·966**
0·45	0·455	0·460	0·465	0·470	0·475	0·480	0·485	0·490	0·495	0·500	0·505	0·510	0·515	0·520	0·525	0·530	0·535	0·540	0·545
	0·060	**0·120**	**0·177**	**0·234**	**0·290**	**0·344**	**0·397**	**0·449**	**0·500**	**0·550**	**0·599**	**0·647**	**0·694**	**0·740**	**0·786**	**0·830**	**0·874**	**0·917**	**0·959**
0·50	0·500	0·500	0·500	0·500	0·500	0·500	0·500	0·500	0·500	0·500	0·500	0·500	0·500	0·500	0·500	0·500	0·500	0·500	0·500
	0·050	**0·100**	**0·150**	**0·200**	**0·250**	**0·300**	**0·350**	**0·400**	**0·450**	**0·500**	**0·550**	**0·600**	**0·650**	**0·700**	**0·750**	**0·800**	**0·850**	**0·900**	**0·950**
0·55	0·545	0·540	0·535	0·530	0·525	0·520	0·515	0·510	0·505	0·500	0·495	0·490	0·485	0·480	0·475	0·470	0·465	0·460	0·455
	0·041	**0·083**	**0·126**	**0·170**	**0·214**	**0·260**	**0·306**	**0·353**	**0·401**	**0·450**	**0·500**	**0·551**	**0·603**	**0·656**	**0·710**	**0·766**	**0·823**	**0·880**	**0·940**
0·60	0·590	0·580	0·570	0·560	0·550	0·540	0·530	0·520	0·510	0·500	0·490	0·480	0·470	0·460	0·450	0·440	0·430	0·420	0·410
	0·034	**0·069**	**0·105**	**0·143**	**0·182**	**0·222**	**0·264**	**0·308**	**0·353**	**0·400**	**0·449**	**0·500**	**0·553**	**0·609**	**0·667**	**0·727**	**0·791**	**0·857**	**0·927**
0·65	0·635	0·620	0·605	0·590	0·575	0·560	0·545	0·530	0·515	0·500	0·485	0·470	0·455	0·440	0·425	0·410	0·395	0·380	0·365
	0·028	**0·056**	**0·087**	**0·119**	**0·152**	**0·188**	**0·225**	**0·264**	**0·306**	**0·350**	**0·397**	**0·447**	**0·500**	**0·557**	**0·618**	**0·683**	**0·753**	**0·829**	**0·911**
0·70	0·680	0·660	0·640	0·620	0·600	0·580	0·560	0·540	0·520	0·500	0·480	0·460	0·440	0·420	0·400	0·380	0·360	0·340	0·320
	0·022	**0·046**	**0·070**	**0·097**	**0·125**	**0·155**	**0·188**	**0·222**	**0·260**	**0·300**	**0·344**	**0·391**	**0·443**	**0·500**	**0·562**	**0·632**	**0·708**	**0·794**	**0·891**
0·75	0·725	0·700	0·675	0·650	0·625	0·600	0·575	0·550	0·525	0·500	0·475	0·450	0·425	0·400	0·375	0·350	0·325	0·300	0·275
	0·017	**0·036**	**0·056**	**0·077**	**0·100**	**0·125**	**0·152**	**0·182**	**0·214**	**0·250**	**0·290**	**0·333**	**0·382**	**0·438**	**0·500**	**0·571**	**0·654**	**0·750**	**0·864**
0·80	0·770	0·740	0·710	0·680	0·650	0·620	0·590	0·560	0·530	0·500	0·470	0·440	0·410	0·380	0·350	0·320	0·290	0·260	0·230
	0·013	**0·027**	**0·042**	**0·059**	**0·077**	**0·097**	**0·119**	**0·143**	**0·170**	**0·200**	**0·234**	**0·273**	**0·317**	**0·368**	**0·429**	**0·500**	**0·586**	**0·692**	**0·826**
0·85	0·815	0·780	0·745	0·710	0·675	0·640	0·605	0·570	0·535	0·500	0·465	0·430	0·395	0·360	0·325	0·290	0·255	0·220	0·185
	0·009	**0·019**	**0·030**	**0·042**	**0·056**	**0·070**	**0·087**	**0·105**	**0·126**	**0·150**	**0·177**	**0·209**	**0·247**	**0·292**	**0·346**	**0·414**	**0·500**	**0·614**	**0·780**
0·90	0·860	0·820	0·780	0·740	0·700	0·660	0·620	0·580	0·540	0·500	0·460	0·420	0·380	0·340	0·300	0·260	0·220	0·180	0·140
	0·006	**0·012**	**0·019**	**0·027**	**0·036**	**0·046**	**0·056**	**0·069**	**0·083**	**0·100**	**0·120**	**0·143**	**0·171**	**0·206**	**0·250**	**0·308**	**0·386**	**0·500**	**0·679**
0·95	0·905	0·860	0·815	0·770	0·725	0·680	0·635	0·590	0·545	0·500	0·455	0·410	0·365	0·320	0·275	0·230	0·185	0·140	0·095
	0·003	**0·006**	**0·009**	**0·013**	**0·017**	**0·022**	**0·028**	**0·034**	**0·041**	**0·050**	**0·060**	**0·073**	**0·089**	**0·109**	**0·136**	**0·174**	**0·220**	**0·321**	**0·500**

The probability that a pair is untied, and therefore provides a preference, is denoted by ϕ, and is given by the formula

$$\phi = \pi_1(1 - \pi_2) + (1 - \pi_1) \pi_2. \qquad (4.1)$$

Table 4.1 gives (in ordinary type) the values of ϕ for various combinations of π_1 and π_2. When π_1 and π_2 are both fairly low, or both fairly

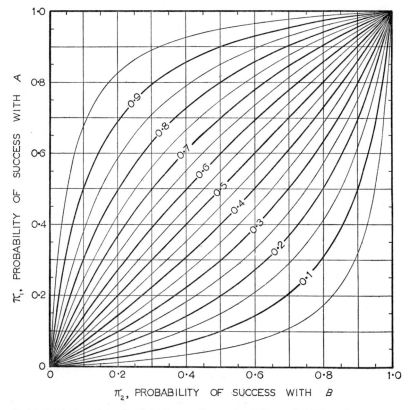

Fig. 4.1. Contour lines for θ in terms of π_1 and π_2, the probabilities of a success with treatments A and B, respectively.

high, ϕ is rather low: most of the pairs are then tied. When either π_1 or π_2 is in the region of $0\cdot5$, ϕ also is about $0\cdot5$: about half the pairs are tied. When π_1 is high and π_2 low (or *vice versa*), ϕ takes fairly high values: most of the pairs are untied. It is one of the characteristic features of this method of forming preferences that we are able to say something about the proportion of paired comparisons which yield usable preferences, whereas, as we have seen in §3.8, this is not so in general.

Of the untied pairs the proportion yielding A preferences, which we denote as usual by θ, is given by

$$\theta = \frac{\pi_1(1 - \pi_2)}{\phi} = \frac{\pi_1(1 - \pi_2)}{\pi_1(1 - \pi_2) + (1 - \pi_1)\,\pi_2}, \qquad (4.2)$$

and the proportion yielding B preferences is

$$1 - \theta = \frac{(1 - \pi_1)\,\pi_2}{\phi} = \frac{(1 - \pi_1)\,\pi_2}{\pi_1(1 - \pi_2) + (1 - \pi_1)\,\pi_2}.$$

The series of preferences is therefore a binomial sequence, the probability of an A preference being θ.

Table 4.1 gives (in bold type) the values of θ corresponding to various combinations of π_1 and π_2, and Fig. 4.1 shows contour lines on which θ takes constant values. The main points to notice are:

(a) when $\pi_1 = \pi_2$, $\theta = \frac{1}{2}$;
(b) when π_1 is greater than π_2, $\theta > \frac{1}{2}$;
(c) when π_1 is less than π_2, $\theta < \frac{1}{2}$;
(d) for a given value of θ, the absolute difference between the probabilities of successes, $\pi_1 - \pi_2$ or $\pi_2 - \pi_1$, is highest when the average of π_1 and π_2 is $\frac{1}{2}$, and decreases as this average approaches 0 or 1. We can put this another way by saying that for a given value of the difference $\pi_1 - \pi_2$ (supposing π_1 to be greater than π_2), θ will be very close to 1 when π_2 is close to zero or when π_1 is close to 1, and will be smallest when the average of π_1 and π_2 is $\frac{1}{2}$. These points are illustrated in Table 4.2.

Table 4.2. Values of θ for various combinations of π_1 and π_2

$\pi_1 - \pi_2 = 0.10$			$\pi_1 - \pi_2 = 0.20$			$\pi_1 - \pi_2 = 0.30$		
π_1	π_2	θ	π_1	π_2	θ	π_1	π_2	θ
0.11	0.01	0.924	0.21	0.01	0.963	0.31	0.01	0.978
0.15	0.05	0.770	0.25	0.05	0.864	0.35	0.05	0.911
0.20	0.10	0.692	0.30	0.10	0.794	0.40	0.10	0.857
0.35	0.25	0.618	0.45	0.25	0.710	0.50	0.20	0.800
0.55	0.45	0.599	0.60	0.40	0.692	0.65	0.35	0.775
0.75	0.65	0.618	0.75	0.55	0.710	0.80	0.50	0.800
0.90	0.80	0.692	0.90	0.70	0.794	0.90	0.60	0.857
0.95	0.85	0.770	0.95	0.75	0.864	0.95	0.65	0.911
0.99	0.89	0.924	0.99	0.79	0.963	0.99	0.69	0.978

It is clear from (a), (b) and (c) that the sequential procedures described in Chapter 3 can be applied to the series of A and B preferences. If the upper boundary is reached, for instance, we have good evidence that $\theta > \frac{1}{2}$, which implies that $\pi_1 > \pi_2$. That is, the probability of success under A is greater than that under B. A path reaching the lower boundary implies that $\pi_2 > \pi_1$, and one reaching the middle boundary means that there is insufficient evidence to say which treatment has the higher probability of success.

Reference is sometimes made in the literature to the *odds ratio*, u, (see, for example, Wald, 1947, Chapter 6). This is defined as follows:

$$u = \frac{\text{Probability of success with } A}{\text{Probability of failure with } A} \div \frac{\text{Probability of success with } B}{\text{Probability of failure with } B}$$

$$= \frac{\pi_1}{1 - \pi_1} \div \frac{\pi_2}{1 - \pi_2} = \frac{\pi_1(1 - \pi_2)}{(1 - \pi_1)\pi_2}.$$

From (4.2), it may be seen that u and θ are connected by the relationships

$$\theta = \frac{u}{1 + u} \quad \text{and} \quad u = \frac{\theta}{1 - \theta}.$$

As θ increases from 0 to 1, u increases from 0 to ∞. When $\theta = \frac{1}{2}$, $u = 1$. It is thus a matter of choice whether the preponderance of A or B preferences is expressed in terms of θ or u.

4.3. The choice of a design

The choice of an open or closed design is available here as in the other situations discussed in Chapter 3. The considerations are essentially the same, and again the closed designs are likely to be the more satisfactory.

Some difficulty may be caused by the fact that the measurements in which one is primarily interested are the probabilities of success, π_1 and π_2, whereas the sequential design is specified in terms of the derived quantity θ. A hypothetical example may perhaps illustrate the way in which the problem can be approached.

Suppose that we are using two methods of administering intravenous drips to post-operative patients, to compare the incidence of thrombophlebitis in each group of patients. From previous experience we might guess the average incidence to be about 30 per cent., or in other words that π_1 and π_2 might be about $0 \cdot 7$ (counting the absence of thrombophlebitis as a success). From Table 4.1, the expected proportion of untied pairs, ϕ, would be about $0 \cdot 4$. As a first statement of the required sensitivity of the trial we might say that if in fact the difference between the incidences is as high as 20 per cent., we should like to have a good chance of detecting the difference. Taking the average of π_1 and π_2 to be 0·7, and making the difference $\pi_1 - \pi_2$ equal to 0·2, would give $\pi_1 = 0·8$, $\pi_2 = 0·6$. From Table 4.1 this would give $\theta = 0·73$, and Table 3.5 shows that for a restricted design with a power of 0·95 of detecting a value $\theta_1 = 0·73$, at a 5 per cent. significance level, we should need a maximum of about $N = 80$ preferences.

Since ϕ is about 0·4, only about 40 per cent. of our pairs of patients will provide usable preferences. The maximum number of pairs of patients required will therefore be about $80/0·4 = 200$; that is, we may require up to about 400 patients. This may be more than would be available within a reasonable period of time, and we may therefore have to revise our requirements. The same sort of calculation may be made for a few different pairs of values of π_1 and π_2, averaging 0·7. The results are shown below:

Difference between π_1 and π_2 to be detected with high probability	π_1	π_2	θ_1	N (approx. from Table 3.5)	Approx. max. no. of pairs $N/(0·4)$
0·1	0·75	0·65	0·62	300	750
0·2	0·80	0·60	0·73	80	200
0·3	0·85	0·55	0·82	34	85
0·4	0·90	0·50	0·90	19	48

We may now feel that only the latter two of these designs would be at all practicable, and we may decide on the restricted procedure with $N = 27$, the boundary points of which are tabulated in Table 3.7.

In this example we have considered pairs of values, π_1 and π_2, with a fixed average. In other situations the investigator may have a fairly reliable idea of the success probability for a standard treatment, but no evidence at all about the value of a new treatment to be compared with it. In this case we could consider a fixed value of π_1 and see what the effect is of varying π_2.

If, as the trial proceeds, it becomes clear that the frequencies of success are much smaller than have been assumed in the preliminary calculations of the type outlined above, it may be necessary to revise the choice of N. Small values of π_1 and π_2 will make ϕ small, and the total number of observations required before N untied pairs are found may be prohibitively large. A reduction in N implies a higher value of θ_1, but an increase in θ_1 may be acceptable if π_1 and π_2 are small, particularly if the investigator wishes to detect a certain absolute difference between π_1 and π_2.

4.4. Confidence limits for $\pi_1 - \pi_2$

In §3.6, we have discussed the setting of confidence limits for θ, when a boundary has been reached and the trial brought to an end. In the present situation the investigator would perhaps be more interested in the difference, $\pi_1 - \pi_2$, between the success probabilities. Again, no theoretical results are available which allow for the sequential design of the investigation, but it will probably be fairly safe to use, as an approximation, the non-sequential result. Suppose that, when the trial stops, there have been r_1 successes with n_1 patients treated by A, and r_2 successes out of n_2 with B. (n_1 and n_2 will be equal if the patients form an exact number of pairs, but may differ a little if some patients are unpaired when the intake stops, or if some results have to be omitted from the analysis for any reason.) Let $r_1/n_1 = p_1$, $r_2/n_2 = p_2$, $q_1 = 1 - p_1$ and $q_2 = 1 - p_2$. Then the standard error of $p_1 - p_2$ is estimated as

$$\sqrt{\left\{ \frac{p_1 q_1}{n_1} + \frac{p_2 q_2}{n_2} \right\}}$$

and approximate 95 per cent. confidence limits for $\pi_1 - \pi_2$ are

$$p_1 - p_2 \pm (2 \times \text{standard error}).$$

As explained in §3.6, if the confidence interval appears to contradict the verdict of the sequential procedure, the latter should be preferred.

4.5. Some examples

Example 4.1

Morrison Smith (1958) investigated the effect of hydrocortisone hemisuccinate as an inhalant for children with asthma. This was a double blind trial, with a placebo preparation indistinguishable from the hydrocortisone and un-identified by the investigators until after the end of the trial. Children were allotted randomly to the two treatment groups, and each child used the speci-fied inhalant daily for a month. The value of the treatment was assessed by respiratory tests at regular intervals and by clinical records, and by collation of the different types of evidence a single judgement was made for each child as to whether treatment had been a 'success' or a 'failure'. Before the trial started it was estimated that 15 per cent. of the children would be likely to benefit by the placebo, and an increase of 50 per cent. in this proportion (i.e. to 65 per cent.) was felt to be sufficiently important to warrant notice. From Table 4.1, the combination $\pi_1 = 0 \cdot 65$ and $\pi_2 = 0 \cdot 15$ gives $\theta = 0 \cdot 913$, and the open design with $\theta_1 = 0 \cdot 90$, $2a = 0 \cdot 05$, $1 - \beta = 0 \cdot 95$ was used (Table 3.1). The middle boundary was crossed at the 6th untied pair. The trial was continued a little longer, by which time 10 untied pairs had been observed and altogether there were 4 successes out of 28 children treated with the placebo and 6 successes out of 29 children treated with hydrocortisone.

Example 4.2

Watkinson (1958) reported a trial to assess the value of hydrocortisone hemi-succinate solution, applied by rectal drip, for patients with mild ulcerative colitis. This treatment was compared with an inert preparation similarly administered. Each patient was treated with one of the two preparations, randomly allocated, for two weeks, and the response of each patient was recorded as a success or failure according to whether remission of symptoms occurred.

The rate of entry of suitable patients into the trial was necessarily rather low, and it was decided to use the restricted design with $2\alpha = 0.05$, $1 - \beta = 0.95$, $\theta_1 = 0.95$, $N = 13$, tabulated in Table 3.7. It was realized that only very striking differences between the proportions of successes would have much chance of being detected by such a small-scale design, but previous uncontrolled studies had suggested that the differences might indeed be considerable.

After 7 pairs of treatment periods* the first boundary point had been reached. There were one tied pair and 6 untied pairs all giving preferences for hydrocortisone. When the results of 5 further treatment periods were added there were 9 remissions out of 10 with hydrocortisone and 1 out of 9 with the placebo.

For a non-sequential trial of the same treatments, see Truelove (1958).

4.6. The use of matched pairs

In the previous sections of this chapter we have assumed that pairing is purely at random, so that there is no correlation between the responses of the two members of a pair. The formulae and tables are, indeed, valid only under this assumption. In §2.5, however, it was suggested that some advantage might be obtained if the population was stratified into sub-groups likely to show some similarity of response, and pairing was carried out within a stratum. The main danger to avoid is an excessive degree of stratification leading to a high proportion of un-paired individuals.

What is the effect of stratification (or *matched pairing*, as it is often called) in a sequential comparison of two proportions? The first point to note is that the proportion of untied pairs, ϕ, is always less than the value given by formula (4.1) which is valid for random pairing. At first sight this might seem a considerable disadvantage, since the analysis is performed on the untied pairs. It is, however, more than compensated for by another effect. For given values of π_1 and π_2, stratification will tend to give a value of θ (the proportion of untied pairs giving A

---

* These involved 13 patients, rather than 14, as one patient had taken part in the trial twice. In the whole investigation, there were 19 treatment periods on 16 patients. The author informs me that some of the details in Tables IV and V of his paper should be modified.

preferences) further away from $\frac{1}{2}$ than would be expected from formula (4.2). This means that, to achieve a high power of detecting a particular difference between π_1 and π_2 we can choose a sequential design with a higher value of θ_1 than would be required for random pairing. This will lead to a reduction in the average number of preferences required and a reduction in the value of N characterizing the restricted procedures. The situation is, then, that we can use a smaller design (i.e. one requiring the use of less preferences), but that preferences are obtained rather less frequently. The combined effect of these two opposing tendencies appears to be beneficial; that is, the advantage seems to lie with the method of matched pairing, as might have been expected. Some results showing that this is so for open designs have been given by Billewicz (1956), but no general results have been proved for restricted designs.

The likely effect of stratification on the maximum sample size in a restricted design will be illustrated by an imaginary example. Suppose two treatments, A and B, are to be compared at the 5 per cent. significance level, in such a way that if the success probabilities are $0\cdot3$ and $0\cdot5$ this difference will be detected with a probability of 95 per cent. Suppose first that the pairing is random. From Table 4.1, this com. bination of success probabilities gives $\theta = 0\cdot70$, and from Table 3.5, this will require a maximum number of preferences, N equal to 104. Table 4.1 shows also that the expected proportion of untied pairs, ϕ, will be $0\cdot5$, and the *expected* maximum number of pairs required will be $104/0\cdot5 = 208.$[*] A similar calculation is shown below on the assumption that both π_1 and π_2 are $0\cdot3$, so that the null hypothesis is satisfied.

	π_1	π_2	θ	ϕ	N	N/ϕ
(i)	$0\cdot5$	$0\cdot3$	$0\cdot70$	$0\cdot50$		208
					104	
(ii)	$0\cdot3$	$0\cdot3$	$0\cdot50$	$0\cdot42$		248

Now, suppose that the population is divided into two strata, and that pairing takes place within the strata. We must postulate some values for the success probabilities in each stratum under conditions (i) and (ii), and these are shown below. If we assume that equal numbers of individuals are drawn from each stratum the success probabilities for the whole populations will be the same as those given above.

---

[*] The actual proportion of untied pairs will not be exactly $\frac{1}{2}$, and there will be some unpredictable variation about 208, which is merely our best guess at the total number of pairs required before 104 untied pairs are found.

SEQUENTIAL MEDICAL TRIALS

	π_1	π_2	θ	Average θ	ϕ	Average ϕ	N	$N/(\text{Av. } \phi)$
(i) Stratum 1	0·3	0·1	0·794		0·34			
				0·738		0·42		176
Stratum 2	0·7	0·5	0·700		0·50			
							74	
(ii) Stratum 1	0·1	0·1	0·500		0·18			
				0·500		0·34		218
Stratum 2	0·5	0·5	0·500		0·50			

The average θ is a weighted average for the two strata. Under conditions (i), for example, untied pairs come less frequently from stratum 1 than from stratum 2 ($\phi = 0·34$ as against $0·50$) and the average θ is

$$\frac{(0·34)\,(0·794) + (0·50)\,(0·700)}{0·34 + 0·50} = 0·738.$$

The maximum number of preferences, N, required to detect a difference giving $\theta = 0·738$ is estimated by graphical interpolation in Table 3.5. The combined effect of the lower values of ϕ and the lower value of N is, as conjectured above, to produce lower values of N/ϕ, the expected maximum number of pairs.

Of course, the values attributed to π_1 and π_2 in such a calculation are no more than rather arbitrary figures for the type of difference which one wishes to detect. The real values might turn out to be quite different. It is in practice difficult to make rational predictions of the effect of stratification on the success probabilities. When stratification is to be used the best approach is probably to plan a trial on the assumption of random pairing. If the stratification is effective the trial may be prolonged somewhat longer than with random pairing, if the treatments do not differ much; but that the power of the experiment has been increased. If the treatments differ appreciably in their effectiveness, the rather slower rate of appearance of untied pairs, with stratification, will probably be largely nullified by the tendency for an outer boundary to be hit after a smaller number of preferences than with random pairing, since θ will be further away from $\frac{1}{2}$.

Billewicz (1958, 1959) has discussed some of the practical aspects of the planning of a sequential trial to assess the effect of body-weight regulation during pregnancy on the incidence and severity of pre-eclampsia. In this trial strict randomization was regarded as impracticable. Women treated in the experimental group were all chosen from one clinic, whereas those in the control group were chosen from other clinics in the same city. For each woman in the experimental group a 'matched pair' in the control group was chosen so that the two resembled each other within defined limits on a number of criteria. The author remarks that previous results suggested that the factors on which matching was based had very little effect on the response, and this impression was confirmed by the results of the trial. Besides the 'matched pair' control, a separate random control was chosen for each woman in the experimental group, and the outcomes of the two sequential comparisons were remarkably similar. In this trial, then, matching probably performed no very useful purpose, but little was lost by doing it. The proportion of unmatchable cases in the experimental group was only 3–4 per cent.

A situation in which matched pairing naturally arises is that in which comparisons are made within subjects. Each subject is observed for two treatment periods, to which A and B are allotted at random. For each period a success or failure is recorded, and the results are treated as in §4.1. The two responses on the same subject are likely to be correlated, probably more highly so than in trials in which different patients are paired within the same stratum.

Cox (1958b) has considered the theory of non-sequential experiments with matched pairs, in which the probabilities of success vary from one pair to another. He shows that the test based on untied pairs alone is an efficient way of detecting departures from the null hypothesis in which the 'odds ratio' is the same for each pair (which implies that θ is the same for each pair).

CHAPTER FIVE

MEASUREMENTS WITH KNOWN VARIABILITY

5.1. Introduction

In the problems considered in previous chapters the response criteria have been qualitative. This limitation is often unavoidable, but there are many situations in which the response is represented by a continuous measurement, or one which assumes, if not a continuous range of values, at least a number of different numerical values. Examples of the latter type of response are frequently encountered in clinical assessments by, say, a 5-point scale. Any measurement, whether continuous or on a scale with a small number of possible values, can always be reduced to a dichotomy. In a 5-point scale, with the values -2, -1, 0, 1 and 2 representing different degrees of clinical change, the scores -2, -1 and 0 can be grouped together as representing no improvement and 1 and 2 as representing some improvement. Example 3.4 describes a trial in which a continuous measurement (the difference between two recovery times) was reduced to a dichotomy by taking account merely of its sign. But any reduction of the scale of measurement involves some loss of information, and methods are required which make use of the recorded value of the measurement, without any arbitrary reduction.

In this and the next chapter we again assume that observations for the two treatments are paired. If no natural pairing is imposed by the design, the pairing is done as usual by random allocation as the trial proceeds. The analysis is performed on the differences between the paired responses, which will be denoted by d. Theoretically these differences are assumed to follow a *normal* distribution, and it is not known to what extent the methods proposed are invalidated by departures from normality. However, it is well known that non-sequential analyses of means of measurements are only slightly affected by moderate departures from normality, and it would be a reasonable conjecture that a similar result holds for sequential analysis. If the distribution of the differences clearly departs widely from normality, a simple transformation of the scale of measurement (say by taking logarithms) may improve matters.

In the present chapter we assume that the variability of the differences (as measured by their standard deviation) is known. This is a very unrealistic assumption, and it is unlikely that the methods will be of much immediate use. They serve, however, as an introduction to those of the next chapter, in which we make no assumption about the variability of the differences. There may occasionally be enough prior information about the variability to justify the use of an assumed value for it.

The analysis is performed on the cumulative sum, y, of the differences, d. The calculation of this sum is illustrated below with some hypothetical measurements:

Pair	Treatment		d	Cumulative sum $y = \Sigma d$
	A	B		
1	6·3	3·7	2·6	2·6
2	4·2	4·4	−0·2	2·4
3	8·4	7·1	1·3	3·7
4	3·7	2·0	1·7	5·4
.	.	.	.	.
.	.	.	.	.
.	.	.	.	.

On the null hypothesis that A and B are equally effective, d should follow a distribution with a mean of zero. If A tends to give higher readings than B, the values of d will tend to be positive; that is, they will follow a distribution with a mean greater than zero. If B tends to give higher readings than A, the mean value of d will be negative. We shall suppose that, whatever the mean of this distribution, the standard deviation is known to be a fixed value, σ. Denote the unknown mean by μ.

As in previous chapters a distinction may be made between open and closed designs, and the methods of procedure for the two types of design are described below. In both cases the designs are characterized by the following properties:

(a) If $\mu = 0$, the probability is about 2α that the sample path reaches one of two outer boundaries, indicating a significant difference between treatments;

(b) if $\mu = \delta_1\sigma$ or $-\delta_1\sigma$ the probability is about $1 - \beta$ that the appropriate outer boundary is reached.

The quantity δ_1 thus plays a similar role to θ_1 in the binomial procedures, indicating the magnitude of difference between treatments which can be detected with a reasonably high power.

5.2. Open designs

The analysis is performed on a chart like that shown in Fig. 5.1. The abscissa is the serial number of the pair, n, and the ordinate is the cumulative sum, $y = \Sigma d$. The equations of the outer boundaries (indicating a significant difference between treatments) are:

$$U : y = \quad a_1\sigma + b\sigma n$$
$$L : y = -a_1\sigma - b\sigma n.$$

The equations of the inner boundaries (indicating no significant difference) are:

$$M \ : y = -a_2\sigma + b\sigma n$$
$$M' : y = \quad a_2\sigma - b\sigma n.$$

As in the binomial design of §3.3 the dotted lines form an extension of the inner boundaries. If the sample path crosses both the dotted lines, the trial stops with no significant difference established.

Table 5.1 gives the values of the constants a_1, a_2 and b, for designs with 5 per cent. significance level ($2\alpha = 0.05$), power $1 - \beta = 0.95$, and for various values of δ_1. Table 5.1 also gives the mean number of pairs needed before a boundary is reached (a) on the null hypothesis that $\mu = 0$, (b) when $\mu = \pm\delta_1\sigma$, and (c) in the most unfavourable circumstances when μ is about $\pm\frac{1}{2}\delta_1$. The number of pairs required for the corresponding non-sequential procedure is also shown. The remarks at the end of §3.3 apply equally well here, and should be re-read.

A possible application of these designs (proposed by van Eeden (1955)), is to compare the proportions of successes with two treatments (the problem considered in Chapter 4). Suppose that observations are made in groups of equal size. The proportion of successes in each group is subjected to the angular transformation, the effect of which is that the differences, d, between the transformed proportions in corres-

Table 5.1. Open sequential designs for normally distributed measurements with known variability. (Two-sided significance level, $2\alpha = 0.05$; power $1 - \beta = 0.95$ at critical value of μ/σ.)

Critical value of μ/σ δ_1	Coefficients in equations of boundaries			Approximate mean number of pairs required			Number of pairs required in equivalent non-sequential procedure
	a_1	a_2	b	(a) when $\mu = 0$	(b) when $\mu = \pm \delta_1\sigma$	(c) at max.	
0·2	18·19	14·85	0·10	205	165	270	325
0·3	12·13	9·90	0·15	91	74	120	145
0·4	9·09	7·43	0·20	51	42	68	82
0·5	7·28	5·94	0·25	33	26	43	52
0·6	6·06	4·95	0·30	23	18	30	37
0·7	5·20	4·24	0·35	17	14	22	27
0·8	4·55	3·71	0·40	13	10	17	21
0·9	4·04	3·30	0·45	10	8	13	17
1·0	3·64	2·97	0·50	8	7	11	13
1·2	3·03	2·48	0·60	6	5	8	10
1·4	2·60	2·12	0·70	4	3	6	7

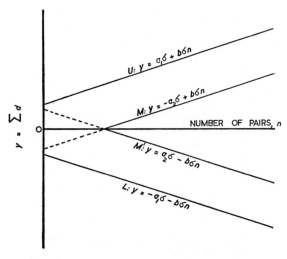

Fig. 5.1. Schematic representation of open design for normally distributed measurements with known variability.

ponding groups have an approximately constant and known standard deviation. For details the paper by van Eeden should be referred to.

An alternative type of 2-sided test is given by Wald (1947, Chapter 9). The relative merits of the alternative methods are not known (see Appendix A.2).

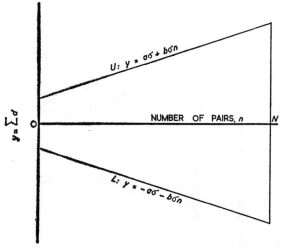

Fig. 5.2. Schematic representation of restricted design for normally distributed measurements with known variability.

Skew designs are obtained by using one pair of parallel lines (either U and M, or L and M').

5.3. Closed designs

The designs described here are 'restricted' procedures similar to those described in §3.4. The abscissa, n, and ordinate, y, of the chart have the same meaning as in the last section. The equations of the outer boundaries are:

$$U : y = \quad a\sigma + b\sigma n$$

$$L : y = -a\sigma - b\sigma n,$$

and the middle boundary, M, consists of a line drawn parallel to the y-axis at $n = N$ (see Fig. 5.2).

Table 5.2. Restricted sequential designs for normally distributed measurements with known variability. (Two-sided significance level, $2\alpha = 0\cdot05$; power $1 - \beta = 0\cdot95$ at critical value of μ/σ.)

Critical value of μ/σ δ_1	Coefficients in equations of boundaries		Maximum number of pairs required N	Number of pairs required in equivalent non-sequential procedure
	a	b		
0·2	18·19	0·10	445	325
0·3	12·13	0·15	198	145
0·4	9·09	0·20	111	82
0·5	7·28	0·25	71	52
0·6	6·06	0·30	49	37
0·7	5·20	0·35	36	27
0·8	4·55	0·40	28	21
0·9	4·04	0·45	22	17
1·0	3·64	0·50	18	13
1·2	3·03	0·60	12	10
1·4	2·60	0·70	9	7

Table 5.2 gives the values of the constants, a, b and N, for designs with $2\alpha = 0\cdot05$, $1 - \beta = 0\cdot95$, and various values of δ_1. The values of a are the same as the corresponding values of a_1 in Table 5.1, and the outer boundaries of the closed and open designs are consequently the same straight lines. The number of pairs required for non-sequential procedures with the same power is also given.

For measurements which have an unlimited range of possible values it is not immediately clear that the middle boundary can be 'collapsed' inwards as in the binomial designs of §3.4, since there is no region to the left of M from which U and L are totally inaccessible. However, if the sample path is progressing towards M in a direction not too much inclined from the horizontal, it becomes more and more unlikely that either U or L will be reached. It should, therefore, be theoretically possible to draw a wedge-shaped middle boundary which would appreciably reduce the number of observations required when the values of y remained low, and at the same time would affect the probabilities of reaching U and L to only a very small extent. This modified middle boundary would not necessarily consist of two straight lines at right angles (as in the binomial designs), and might instead be curved. Similarly, skew closed designs, similar in shape to those of Fig. 3.9, could be obtained. Detailed results are not yet available.

CHAPTER SIX

MEASUREMENTS WITH UNKNOWN VARIABILITY

6.1. Introduction

The methods of Chapter 5 are of limited value, because the variability of the observations, as measured by the standard deviation, σ, of the differences, is assumed to be known. One may frequently have some preliminary evidence about σ which will be useful in planning the trial, but it will usually be unsafe to rely on this estimate of σ in the analysis. Exactly the same situation arises in non-sequential statistical analyses. In comparing two means by calculating the standard error of their difference, one would not normally evaluate this standard error in terms of some preconceived value for the standard deviation of the individual observations. This standard deviation would be estimated from the results themselves, and the ratio of the difference between the means to its standard error would be referred to tables of the t-distribution.

Similarly, then, in the sequential analysis of an experiment to compare two treatments, the relevant random variability should be estimated from the observations themselves. The resulting test is known as a *sequential t-test*.

In an experiment yielding a series of differences, as in §5.1, the orthodox non-sequential procedure is to calculate a quantity, t, which is the ratio of the mean difference to an estimate of its standard error (Moroney, 1956, Chapter 13; Bailey, 1959, §6.2). It would be possible to perform the sequential analysis by calculating t at each stage (see Armitage, 1954) but this would be rather tedious. An equivalent, but much simpler, procedure is to calculate at each stage a quantity, z, given by the formula

$$z = \frac{(\Sigma d)^2}{\Sigma d^2}.$$

Here Σd is the cumulative sum of differences for all the pairs so far recorded, and Σd^2 is the cumulative sum of the squares of these differences. For the example of §5.1 the calculations would proceed as follows:

Pair	A	B	d	d^2	Σd	$(\Sigma d)^2$	Σd^2	z
1	6·3	3·7	2·6	6·76	2·6	6·76	6·76	1·00
2	4·2	4·4	−0·2	0·04	2·4	5·76	6·80	0·85
3	8·4	7·1	1·3	1·69	3·7	13·69	8·49	1·61
4	3·7	2·0	1·7	2·89	5·4	29·16	11·38	2·56

On the null hypothesis, the values of d come from a population whose mean, μ, is zero, and z will tend to remain fairly low. If A tends to give higher, or lower, readings than B, d will tend to increase, with either a positive or a negative sign, and z also will tend to increase. Note that since z is calculated in terms of $(\Sigma d)^2$, the sign of Σd does not affect the value of z, which is always positive.

As before, we denote the standard deviation of the distribution of d by σ. This measures the variability of d in an infinitely long random sequence, and is not known exactly. An estimate of σ from a finite number of pairs (e.g. from the four values of d given in the example above) may be either less or greater than the true value, since the d's will vary randomly and unpredictably.

We shall again make a distinction between open and closed designs. The types of boundaries used are described in detail below. In both cases the designs have the following properties:

(a) If $\mu = 0$, the probability is about 2α that the sample path reaches the outer boundary, indicating a significant difference;

(b) if $\mu = \delta_1\sigma$ or $-\delta_1\sigma$ the probability is about $1 - \beta$ that the outer boundary is reached.

These properties are essentially the same as those of §5.1, but the essential difference in interpretation is that σ was then supposed to be known whereas here it is unknown. Since the designs are specified in terms of δ_1 and σ is unknown, it follows that for a particular design $\delta_1\sigma$ is unknown. This means that the magnitude of the mean difference which can be detected with a given power is unknown. This may seem surprising, but a little reflection shows that it would be expected. The sensitivity of a specified design must depend on the variability of the observations. If this is high, then only very large differences between treatments will be detected. If successive observations are very uniform, the experiment will be able to detect relatively small effects.

If prior information is available about σ, this may enable the investigator to make a reasonable guess at the value of $\delta_1 \sigma$ for any particular design; or, conversely, to choose a value of δ_1 (and hence a design) so that he has a good chance of detecting a particular mean difference, $\mu = \delta_1 \sigma$. In the absence of any relevant prior information, one approach would be to collect a sufficient number of observations to provide an estimate of σ, before finally deciding on the sequential design.

6.2. Open designs

The procedure is to plot the successive values of z on a chart like that of Fig. 6.1. The upper boundary, U, indicates a significant difference in either direction, and the lower boundary, M, indicates that no significant difference has been found. This type of chart is essentially different from those presented previously. Whereas in previous charts there have been two outer boundaries representing differences in either direction, their functions are now combined by the single upper boundary, U. If a path reaches U it will, of course, be perfectly clear from the sign of d in which direction the difference lies. We denote the lower boundary by M, rather than L, to emphasize that it corresponds to the inner boundaries M and M' in the open designs of §§3.3 and 5.2.

The boundary points for each value of n are given in the National Bureau of Standards tables (1951). We shall refer to this publication as the 'N.B.S. tables'. In these tables the critical value δ_1 is referred to as δ, and tables are presented for values of δ at intervals of $0 \cdot 1$ up to $1 \cdot 0$, at intervals of $0 \cdot 2$ to $2 \cdot 0$, and also the value $2 \cdot 5$. The headings to the columns of each table are the values* of $\ln\{(1 - \beta)/2\alpha\}$ for U, and $-\ln\{(1 - 2\alpha)/\beta\}$ for M. The columns most useful for our present purposes are those headed 'ln 19' and '$-$ln 19' which refer to U and M, respectively, when $2\alpha = \beta = 0 \cdot 05$; and those headed 'ln 99' and '$-$ln 99' which correspond to $2\alpha = \beta = 0 \cdot 01$.

The N.B.S. tables should be referred to for full details of the boundaries, but an abridged table for the case $2\alpha = \beta = 0 \cdot 05$ is given in Table 6.1. The boundaries are for the most part very nearly straight lines, and if necessary can be extended linearly at the right-hand end (i.e. for large values of n). The upper boundary is initially curved, as

---

* ln denotes the natural or Naperian logarithm, to base e.

*Table 6.1.*Sequential *t*-test (open design) with $2\alpha = 0.05$; $1 - \beta = 0.95$. The tabulated quantities are the values of z on the boundaries. The upper number of each pair refers to the upper boundary, U, and the lower number to the lower boundary, L. (From tables published by the National Bureau of Standards (1951).)

Number of observations, n

Critical value of δ_1	20	40	60	80	100	120	140	160	180	200
0·2	18·94 / —	11·80 / —	9·45 / —	8·35 /	7·76 /	7·44 /	7·26 /	7·17 / 0·09	7·15 / 0·22	7·17 / 0·37
0·3	10·51 / —	7·78 / —	7·12 / —	7·00 / 0·22	7·10 / 0·55	7·32 / 0·91	7·59 / 1·29	7·91 / 1·68	8·26 / 2·08	8·62 / 2·49
0·4	7·75 / —	6·81 / 0·09	6·98 / 0·66	7·45 / 1·32	8·03 / 2·02	8·68 / 2·74	9·36 / 3·47	10·06 / 4·22	10·79 / 4·97	11·52 / 5·72
0·5	6·68 / —	6·81 / 0·74	7·62 / 1·77	8·60 / 2·87	9·69 / 4·00	10·78 / 5·15	11·91 / 6·31			
0·6	6·29 / 0·22	7·26 / 1·62	8·67 / 3·18	10·18 / 4·80	11·76 / 6·43					

Number of observations, n

Critical value of δ_1	5	10	15	20	25	30	35	40	45	50
0·7	— / —	6·03 / —	6·01 / 0·25	6·25 / 0·68	6·61 / 1·16	7·03 / 1·66	7·49 / 2·17	7·96 / 2·69	8·46 / 3·21	8·96 / 3·74
0·8	— / —	5·65 / 0·09	5·94 / 0·64	6·41 / 1·25	6·97 / 1·89	7·57 / 2·54	8·19 / 3·21	8·83 / 3·88	9·48 / 4·56	10·14 / 5·24
0·9	— / —	5·46 / 0·37	6·01 / 1·10	6·69 / 1·88	7·44 / 2·69	8·21 / 3·51	9·01 / 4·33	9·81 / 5·16	10·63 / 6·00	11·44 / 6·83
1·0	4·98 / —	5·39 / 0·69	6·16 / 1·61	7·05 / 2·57	7·97 / 3·54	8·92 / 4·52	9·88 / 5·51	10·85 / 6·50		
1·2	4·48 / 0·22	5·45 / 1·42	6·63 / 2·70	7·88 / 4·00	9·16 / 5·30	10·45 / 6·62				
1·4	4·23 / 0·61	5·64 / 2·19	7·20 / 3·80	8·79 / 5·42	10·39 / 7·05					

Critical value of δ_1	Values at start of U n	Values at start of U z	Value of n at lowest point of U	Equivalent fixed-sample size, N_0
0·2	20	18·94	181	327
0·3	14	12·94	78	147
0·4	11	10·00	43	85
0·5	9	8·34	27	54
0·6	8	7·14	18	39
0·7	7	6·37	13	29
0·8	6	5·83	9	23
0·9	6	5·32	7	19
1·0	5	4·98	5	16
1·2	5	4·48	5	12
1·4	4	4·00	4	

illustrated in Fig. 6.1. Note that this boundary is initially not defined until a certain minimum number of pairs has been observed. For example, in the design with $\delta_1 = 1$, the upper boundary cannot be reached until at least 5 pairs have been observed. The lower boundary in this design starts at the 6th pair.

A numerical illustration of this type of sequential procedure is given by Hajnal, Sharp and Popert (1959). In the next section we describe in detail an example of the rather similar procedure for closed designs.

A number of alternative methods of performing sequential t-tests

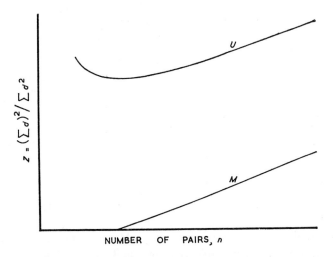

Fig. 6.1. Schematic representation of open design for normally distributed measurements with unknown variability (sequential t-test).

have been proposed (see Appendix A.2). The two-sided test described by Davies (1954) differs slightly from that presented here, being rather more analogous to the previous open designs of §§3.3 and 5.2, in having two separate open channels. The relative merits of different proposals are not yet entirely clear, but the method described here has the advantage of using the excellent and extensive N.B.S. tables. Rushton (1952) describes a method of performing the present test which is useful for situations beyond the range covered by the N.B.S. tables.

Rushton (1952) describes the sequential t-test appropriate if the observations in the two series are not paired. This is probably somewhat more efficient than the pairing method proposed here, although one would expect there to be very little gain in fairly large experiments. The procedure can be carried out by means of the N.B.S. tables, although a certain amount of interpolation is necessary. The advantage of pairing has already been discussed in §2.5.

Example 6.1

Hajnal, Sharp and Popert (1959) used open sequential t-tests to compare the relative efficacies of different analgesics for patients with rheumatoid arthritis. Patients were treated in successive weeks by each of two drugs, the order of administration being reversed for alternate patients. Each patient's performance was measured three times a week by his score on a grip test, and the basic observation, d, was the sum of the difference between the mean scores in successive weeks for a patient receiving the drugs in the order AB, and the corresponding difference for the next patient, for whom the order was BA.

The critical difference, δ_1, was chosen to be $0 \cdot 85$. This was believed to be rather smaller than the difference between aspirin and a placebo. Three trials are reported. In the first, prednisone was shown to be better than aspirin (at least, by the chosen criterion) after 7 values of d (that is, after two-weekly treatment periods on 14 patients). In the second trial, no significant difference was detected between phenylbutazone and aspirin (the trial stopping after 13 pairs of patients). The third trial showed aspirin to be better than N-acetyl-para-aminophenol (N.A.P.A.P.) after 29 pairs (cf. Ex. 3.2).

This paper contains an interesting discussion of the advantages and difficulties associated with sequential trials.

6.3. Closed designs

As in the situations described in §§3.4 and 5.3, a restricted procedure can be obtained from the open design by retaining the outer boundary U, and re-drawing the lower boundary, M, as a line parallel to the z-axis at $n = N$. An example is shown in Fig. 6.2. The theoretical problem of determining N is unsolved, but the values given in Table 6.1 should provide a satisfactory approximation. The quantities N_0 given in Table 6.1 are the numbers of differences required by the relevant non-sequential procedures. The basis of the approximation for N is that the ratio N/N_0 is given the value of $1 \cdot 37$, which is appropriate when σ is known (Armitage, 1957). The accuracy of this approximation is uncertain, but one would conjecture that the error is likely to be no greater than that due to non-normality of the observations. The method by which the upper boundary is determined ensures that whatever value is chosen for N the probability of reaching U when the null hypothesis is true is less than $1/19 = 0 \cdot 053$, and for the values of N thus calculated the probability should be close to its nominal value of $0 \cdot 05$.

Example 6.2

To illustrate a closed sequential t-test, we consider the data used by Robertson and Armitage (1959) in the trial of two hypotensive agents described in

Example 3.4. For purposes of comparison with the previous analysis based on preferences we again choose a procedure with $N = 62$. From the approximation given above, this corresponds to a non-sequential procedure with $N_0 = 62/1\cdot37 = 45$, for which $\delta_1 = 0\cdot55$, as may be checked roughly from Table 6.1. The appropriate boundary points are found by interpolation from the N.B.S. tables, and the boundaries are drawn in Fig. 6.2.

The recovery times observed in the trial, and the differences of the paired values, are given in Table 6.2, which shows the details of the computation of the successive values of z. The path formed by plotting these values on the chart is shown in Fig. 6.2. The path rose rather sharply to $n = 12$, corresponding to the downward trend of the preferences in Fig. 3.8. Subsequently

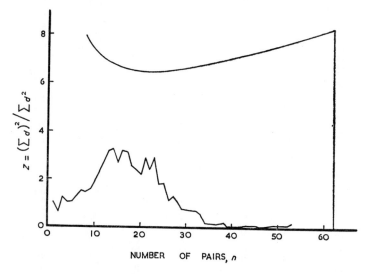

Fig. 6.2. Closed sequential t-test, exemplified by data from Table 6.2.
$(2a = 0\cdot05, 1 - \beta = 0\cdot95, \delta_1 = 0\cdot55, N = 62.)$

the values of z fell gradually and the 'non-significant' boundary would almost certainly have been reached at $n = 62$. Only 53 pairs of patients took part in the trial, however. In the analysis by preferences the middle boundary, which points inwards, was reached at $n = 49$. One more pair entered the trial, and three pairs provided no preference, making 53 in all. In the analysis by preferences one could say at $n = 49$ that the outer boundaries could not possibly be reached with the maximum of 62 pairs. In the sequential t-test this event cannot entirely be precluded but it is clear from Fig. 6.2 that the path would be very unlikely to turn suddenly upwards and hit the upper boundary.

The extra power obtained by using measurements rather than preferences is shown by the fact that the critical value $\theta_1 = 0\cdot75$, which could be detected with a power of $0\cdot95$ in the analysis by preferences, would correspond to a mean difference, $\mu = 0\cdot67\sigma$, provided the differences were normally distri-

6

buted. The sequential t-test, as we have seen, has the same power of detecting a mean difference, $\mu = 0\cdot55\sigma$, a considerably smaller contrast between the treatments.

Table 6.2. Calculations for sequential t-test (Example 6·2).

Pair	Recovery time (mins.) for patient treated with		Difference d	Σd	Σd^2	z
	Phen. chlor.	Trimet.				
1	102	7	95	95	9,025	1·00
2	6	26	−20	75	9,425	0·60
3	57	16	41	116	11,106	1·21
4	13	23	−10	106	11,206	1·00
5	8	7	1	107	11,207	1·02
6	23	11	12	119	11,351	1·25
7	26	15	11	130	11,472	1·47
8	8	10	−2	128	11,476	1·43
9	14	8	6	134	11,512	1·56
10	22	8	14	148	11,708	1·87
11	37	18	19	167	12,069	2·31
12	75	4	71	238	17,110	3·31
13	5	14	−9	229	17,191	3·05
14	17	10	7	236	17,240	3·23
15	27	46	−19	217	17,601	2·68
16	36	13	23	240	18,130	3·18
17	17	21	−4	236	18,146	3·07
18	19	39	−20	216	18,546	2·52
19	17	24	−7	209	18,595	2·35
20	3	12	−9	200	18,676	2·14
21	49	9	40	240	20,276	2·84
22	9	28	−19	221	20,637	2·37
23	36	12	24	245	21,213	2·83
24	22	65	−43	202	23,062	1·77
25	20	20	0	202	23,062	1·77
26	22	60	−38	164	24,506	1·10
27	21	12	9	173	24,587	1·22
28	12	25	−13	160	24,756	1·03
29	21	45	−24	136	25,332	0·73
30	28	31	−3	133	25,341	0·70
31	3	10	−7	126	25,390	0·63
32	24	23	1	127	25,391	0·64
33	8	22	−14	113	25,587	0·50
34	5	60	−55	58	28,612	0·12
35	22	22	0	58	28,612	0·12
36	4	21	−17	41	28,901	0·06
37	19	13	6	47	28,937	0·08
38	27	14	13	60	29,106	0·12
39	22	72	−50	10	31,606	0·00
40	25	25	0	10	31,606	0·00
41	20	28	−8	2	31,670	0·00
42	6	4	2	4	31,674	0·00
43	30	10	20	24	32,074	0·02
44	16	9	7	31	32,123	0·03
45	14	27	−13	18	32,292	0·01
46	13	50	−37	−19	33,661	0·01
47	45	26	19	0	34,022	0
48	4	25	−21	−21	34,463	0·01
49	14	28	−14	−35	34,659	0·04
50	9	12	−3	−38	34,668	0·04
51	2	11	−9	−47	34,749	0·06
52	16	8	8	−39	34,813	0·04
53	7	44	−37	−76	36,182	0·16

Example 6.2 suggests that some indentation of the middle boundary could theoretically be achieved without any appreciable effect on the probabilities of hitting the upper boundary. The theoretical solution to this problem will probably not be available until the corresponding problem for known variability has been solved (see §5.3). The solution to the latter problem could then be used as an approximation for the more realistic situation considered in the present chapter.

6.4. Skew designs

Open skew designs, for one-sided sequential t-tests, have been described by Rushton (1950) and Davies (1954). Tables computed by Rushton are included in Davies's book. Details are not given here, but it will suffice to remark that the procedure involves the computation of z, defined as in §6.1, but that the boundaries are defined in terms of $\sqrt{z}$, which is given the same sign as its numerator, Σd. There are two boundaries, one indicating a significant advantage of one treatment, say A, over the other, and the other boundary indicating no significant advantage to A.

Example 6.3

Kilpatrick and Oldham (1954) describe two trials, designed to detect a possible advantage of calcium chloride over adrenaline as a bronchial dilator. Each subject received inhalations of the two substances, in a random order, and the expiratory flow rate was measured before and after each inhalation. Denoting the gain in expiratory flow rate after each inhalation (as compared with the reading before inhalation) by g, the difference between the two values of g is the basic variate d.

The boundaries were chosen to give a (one-sided) significance level $a = 0.01$, and a power $1 - \beta = 0.99$ with respect to a value of $\delta_1 = 1$ (representing a possible advantage to calcium chloride. In each trial only 4 values of d (i.e. 4 subjects) were required before the boundary indicating no significant advantage to calcium chloride was reached. As it happened, all the 8 values of d (4 from each trial) had the same sign (favouring adrenaline), so there is a strong supposition that calcium chloride was inferior to adrenaline. Unfortunately, it is theoretically difficult to perform a two-sided test with a one-sided design, and this question remained unresolved.

Skew restricted designs for sequential t-tests are not yet available, and will presumably be available only when the corresponding problem for known variability has been solved, and its solution can be used as an approximation when the variability is unknown.

6.5. The number of observations required

Table 6.1 gives no details about the mean number of observations required to reach a boundary, for either open or closed designs. Hardly anything is known theoretically about the distribution of the number of observations, but one would conjecture that, for open designs with a particular value δ_1, the mean number of observations required in a sequential t-test would be slightly greater than that required when σ is known. Some values appropriate to the latter case are given in Table 5.1.

CHAPTER SEVEN

FOLLOW-UP STUDIES

7.1. General considerations

The principal point to be made here has already been discussed briefly in §2.4 (i).

In a sequential analysis observations are subjected to continuous scrutiny as they become available. It is evident, therefore, that a sequential analysis will be most effective if the observations are made rapidly, so that a decision to stop, resulting from the analysis of a certain number of observations, can be put into effect before many more subjects have been treated. Many therapeutic procedures, on the other hand, must be evaluated by responses which become available after a relatively long period of time. The follow-up period will usually have a fixed duration (for example, radiographic assessments may be made one year after treatment), but may be variable, as in the measurement of survival time, the duration of remission of symptoms, or the duration of occurrence of symptoms.

The possible benefit of a sequential analysis depends, broadly, on the relative magnitudes of the response time (the time elapsing between a particular application of a treatment and the time at which the response is available), and the maximum length of intake of subjects into the trial. As an illustration, suppose that subjects become available for treatment at an even rate of 100 pairs each year, and that the maximum length of intake is precisely one year.* Table 7.1 shows, for various alternative values of the response-time, the possible reduction in the number of observations which could be achieved by using a restricted design permitting closure before the year's intake had stopped. For example, if the response-time is 0·6 years, the first results will not become available until the intake is more than half completed, and total number of pairs used can range only from 60 to 100. Furthermore, the sequential procedure which might permit this reduction below 100

---

* A year is used here as an arbitrary time unit. The argument would be equally valid if 'years' were replaced by 'months'.

pairs can itself be based on a maximum of $N = 40$ pairs. The longer the response time, the smaller the value of N, and the less powerful will be the sequential procedure.

Table 7.1. Possible reduction in observations for trial with intake of 100 pairs a year, for maximum period of one year.

Response-time	Maximum number of pairs available for sequential analysis	Minimum number of pairs in trial
0·2	80	20
0·4	60	40
0·6	40	60
0·8	20	80

In general, then, it is hardly worth considering the application of sequential procedures if the intake period is definitely limited, and if the response-time normally is much more than half the maximum intake period.

In the trial described by Billewicz (1958, 1959), discussed earlier in §4.6, women were treated early in pregnancy, and there was necessarily a delay of up to 7 months between the start of treatment for any woman and the time at which the response was measured. Nevertheless, this delay time was short in comparison with the length of the intake period. The trial was originally planned as an open binomial design, with an expected duration of 3 to 4 years' intake.

For studies in which the response is available after a fixed follow-up period there is no special problem about the sequential analysis, which, may, according to the type of response, follow any of the methods described in earlier chapters. Even where the follow-up period varies (as it does to a very minor extent, for instance, in the pregnancy study described above), it may be more convenient to wait a fixed period after treatment before using each observation. In the next section, however, we consider a type of study in which the follow-up period may vary very considerably, and in which the period elapsing between treatment and analysis is not fixed.

7.2. The comparison of response times

In some trials the main question is whether certain treatments differ in their effects on the time elapsing before a certain response is observed. In malignant disease, for example, it might be asked whether one treatment tends to lengthen survival time as compared with another treatment. In diseases with a pattern of alternating remissions and relapses, such as disseminated sclerosis or ulcerative colitis, the aim might be to detect an increase in the duration of a remission. For patients recovering from a particular disease the object might be to shorten the period during which symptoms are experienced.

If the complete duration of the trial is likely to be much longer than any of the individual response times, this situation could be approached by the methods of Chapter 6. Patients would be paired on entry to the trial, and for each pair the difference in length between the two response times would be calculated and would form the basis of a sequential *t*-test. Such differences cannot, of course, be calculated until the *longer* of the two response times has been completed. On the other hand, some sort of comparative information is clearly available as soon as the *shorter* time is completed. For example, if a patient on treatment *A* has a response time of 3 days and the response time for a patient treated at the same time with *B* is 6 weeks, we do not need to wait 6 weeks before saying that for this pair *A* appears to be better (or worse, according to the type of response) than *B*. At the first response, 3 days after treatment, we can immediately score a qualitative preference for *A* or *B*. Some information is, of course, wasted by ignoring the exact response times, or the magnitude of their difference, but this is partially counteracted by the earlier availability of the observations. Such a comparison has been called the *sign method* (Armitage, 1958*b*; 1959), because it is based on the signs of the differences between paired response times and not on their magnitudes.

If, as must invariably be true, the two patients forming a pair are not treated at exactly the same time, each patient's response time must be measured from the time of his own treatment. It may then happen that the first response to occur does not correspond to the shorter response time. An illustration of the way in which preferences are recorded is shown in Fig. 7.1. The number of preferences recorded at any stage is always less than the number of pairs of patients already treated. It should also be noted that the preferences provided by the various pairs do not, in general, become available in the same order as that in which the pairs are treated.

It will be convenient, from now onwards, to think of the response as being death, so that the object of treatment is to *lengthen* the response times. The proportion of survivors, when plotted against the time after treatment, is called the *survival curve*. It must be emphasized, however, that the methods described here are applicable for a wide variety of responses, as indicated in the first paragraph of this section.

If the null hypothesis, that the two treatments are equally effective, is true, and assuming as usual that treatments are allocated randomly to the two members of each pair, then preferences for A or B will clearly be equally likely. That is, the preferences will form a binomial sequence in which the probability of an A preference, θ, is equal to $\frac{1}{2}$.

It is also fairly clear that if A is better than B, in the sense that the survival curve for A is, on the average, higher than that for B, then θ will be greater than $\frac{1}{2}$. Similarly, if B is in this sense better than A, θ

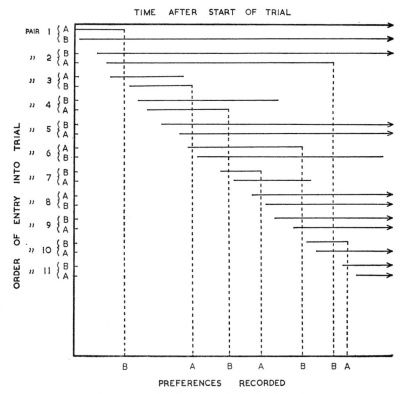

Fig. 7.1. Example of use of the sign method. The horizontal lines represent the periods of survival of different patients and the vertical lines show when the preferences are obtained.

will be less than $\frac{1}{2}$. We have, then, the type of situation already discussed in Chapter 3, and a natural proposal would be to use the same sequential methods.

Now, the sequential procedures described in Chapter 3 are defined by the risks of error, α and β, and by the value of θ, called θ_1, which we wish to be able to detect. An important problem, then, is to interpret the quantity θ in terms of the differences between the survival curves.

A second point to be examined is the relationship between N (the maximum number of preferences required in a restricted design) and the maximum number of patients, which will, of course, be greater than N.

If the null hypothesis is not true, it does not necessarily follow that the preferences will follow a binomial sequence with a constant value of θ. Suppose, for instance, that the survival curves crossed over, as in Fig. 7.2. Preferences arising very early in the trial would be determined

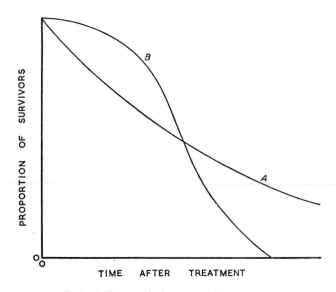

Fig. 7.2. Two survival curves which cross over.

by the initial portions of the survival curves, and (in the example of Fig. 7.2) θ would be less than $\frac{1}{2}$. In due course, however, the preferences would be determined by the later, as well as the earlier, parts of the curves, and θ might rise above $\frac{1}{2}$. It can be shown that the preferences will form a binomial sequence with constant θ if and only if the proportion of survivors at any particular time after treatment, under A, is obtained by raising the survival proportion under B to a constant power, k. When this happens, $\theta = 1/(1 + k)$. Suppose, for example, that the survival proportion under A is the square of that under B. Then $k = 2$, and $\theta = 1/3$. If the rôles of A and B are interchanged, $k = \frac{1}{2}$ and $\theta = 2/3$.

It must be stressed that although this requirement is rather rigid, and is perhaps unlikely to be exactly fulfilled in practice, the sign method is by no means invalidated. The situation we have described, which leads to a constant θ, is merely one sort of alternative to the null hypothesis which it is possible to consider and to guard against. If the survival curves differ sufficiently greatly, even though the series of preferences does not yield a constant θ, the A's or the B's will predominate and an outer boundary will have a good chance of being reached. This point has already been discussed in relation to preferences in general (§3.1).

The 'constant-power' relationship between survival curves does, in

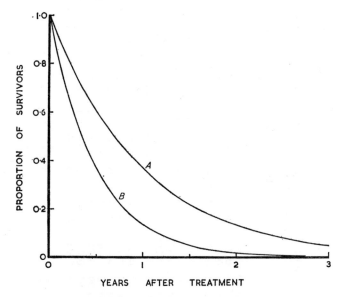

Fig. 7.3. Exponential survival curves with $\lambda_A = 1$, $\lambda_B = 2$.

fact, hold for one of the simplest theoretical types of survival curve— the exponential. Suppose that, in successive time-intervals of a fixed length, a constant proportion of the surviving population dies. The resulting survival curve may be written in the form

$P(t)$ (= Proportion of survivors at time t after treatment)
$\quad = e^{-\lambda t}$.

The quantity λ measures the steepness of the survival curve, and determines the mean survival time after treatment, which is $1/\lambda$. If both

Table 7.2. Proportion of survivors at time t after treatment, for an exponential curve, $e^{-\lambda t}$.

t λ	0·2	0·4	0·6	0·8	1·0	1·2	1·4	1·6	1·8	2·0	2·5	3·0
0·2	0·96	0·92	0·89	0·85	0·82	0·79	0·76	0·73	0·70	0·67	0·61	0·55
0·4	0·92	0·85	0·79	0·73	0·67	0·62	0·57	0·53	0·49	0·45	0·37	0·30
0·6	0·89	0·79	0·70	0·62	0·55	0·49	0·43	0·38	0·34	0·30	0·22	0·17
0·8	0·85	0·73	0·62	0·53	0·45	0·38	0·33	0·28	0·24	0·20	0·14	0·09
1·0	0·82	0·67	0·55	0·45	0·37	0·30	0·25	0·20	0·17	0·14	0·08	0·05
1·2	0·79	0·62	0·49	0·38	0·30	0·24	0·19	0·15	0·12	0·09	0·05	0·03
1·4	0·76	0·57	0·43	0·33	0·25	0·19	0·14	0·11	0·08	0·06	0·03	0·01
1·6	0·73	0·53	0·38	0·28	0·20	0·15	0·11	0·08	0·06	0·04	0·02	0·01
1·8	0·70	0·49	0·34	0·24	0·17	0·12	0·08	0·06	0·04	0·03	0·01	0·00
2·0	0·67	0·45	0·30	0·20	0·14	0·09	0·06	0·04	0·03	0·02	0·01	0·00
2·5	0·61	0·37	0·22	0·14	0·08	0·05	0·03	0·02	0·01	0·01	0·00	0·00
3·0	0·55	0·30	0·17	0·09	0·05	0·03	0·01	0·01	0·00	0·00	0·00	0·00
3·5	0·50	0·25	0·12	0·06	0·03	0·01	0·01	0·00	0·00	0·00	0·00	0·00
4·0	0·45	0·20	0·09	0·04	0·02	0·01	0·00	0·00	0·00	0·00	0·00	0·00
4·5	0·41	0·17	0·07	0·03	0·01	0·00	0·00	0·00	0·00	0·00	0·00	0·00
5·0	0·37	0·14	0·05	0·02	0·01	0·00	0·00	0·00	0·00	0·00	0·00	0·00

Table 7.3. Values of G, the average number of preferences obtained at a time T after the start of the trial, in terms of mT (the number of pairs entered by time T) and $\bar{\lambda}T$ ($\bar{\lambda}$ being the mean of the constants defining the two exponential curves.)

mT \ $\bar{\lambda}T$	0·1	0·2	0·3	0·4	0·5	0·6	0·7	0·8	0·9	1·0	1·2	1·4	1·6	1·8	2·0	3·0	4·0	5·0	∞
20	2	4	5	6	7	8	9	10	11	11	12	13	14	15	15	17	18	18	20
40	4	7	10	12	15	17	18	20	21	23	25	27	28	29	30	33	35	36	40
60	6	11	15	19	22	25	28	30	32	34	37	40	42	44	45	50	53	54	60
80	7	14	20	25	29	33	37	40	43	45	50	53	56	58	60	67	70	72	80
100	9	18	25	31	37	42	46	50	54	57	62	66	70	73	75	83	88	90	100
120	11	21	30	37	44	50	55	60	64	68	75	80	84	88	91	100	105	108	120
140	13	25	35	44	52	58	65	70	75	79	87	93	98	102	106	117	123	126	140
160	15	28	40	50	59	67	74	80	86	91	99	106	112	117	121	133	140	144	160
180	17	32	45	56	66	75	83	90	97	102	112	120	126	131	136	150	158	162	180
200	19	35	50	62	74	84	92	100	107	114	124	133	140	146	151	167	175	180	200
250	23	44	62	78	92	104	115	125	134	142	155	166	175	182	189	208	219	225	250
300	28	53	74	93	110	125	139	150	161	170	186	199	210	219	226	250	263	270	300
350	33	62	87	109	129	146	162	175	188	199	217	233	245	255	264	292	306	315	350
400	37	70	99	125	147	167	185	200	215	227	248	266	280	292	302	334	350	360	400
450	42	79	112	140	166	188	208	226	241	255	280	299	315	328	340	375	394	405	450
500	47	88	124	156	184	209	231	251	268	284	311	332	350	365	377	417	438	450	500

A and B lead to exponential survival curves, their formulae may be written

$$P_A(t) = e^{-\lambda_A t}$$

and

$$P_B(t) = e^{-\lambda_B t}$$

$$\left. \right\} \qquad (7.1)$$

From these expressions it follows that $P_A(t) = \{P_B(t)\}^{(\lambda_A/\lambda_B)}$. That is, $k = \lambda_A/\lambda_B$, and the preferences will follow a binomial sequence with $\theta = 1/(1 + k) = \lambda_B/(\lambda_A + \lambda_B)$.

Fig. 7.3 illustrates two survival curves with time measured in years, for which $\lambda_A = 1$ and $\lambda_B = 2$. Survival curves will not always approximate to the exponential form, but this type of curve has frequently been proposed as an adequate representation of actual observations and will probably provide a rough approximation in most instances. The values of the proportion of survivors, for various values of the time t and the parameter λ, are given in Table 7.2.

Suppose that patients are admitted to the trial at a uniform rate of m per unit time to each of two treatments, A and B; and that the survival curves are given by (7.1). Then the number of preferences which would be obtained, on the average, by a time T after the start of the trial is

$$G = mT\left\{1 - \frac{1 - e^{-2\bar{\lambda}T}}{2\bar{\lambda}T}\right\}, \qquad (7.2)$$

where $\bar{\lambda} = \frac{1}{2}(\lambda_A + \lambda_B)$. This number, G, is, of course, necessarily less than mT (the number of pairs of patients entered into the trial) since not all these pairs will have provided preferences by the time T. Note that G depends not on λ_A and λ_B separately, but on their average, $\bar{\lambda}$. Table 7.3 gives the values of G, for various values of mT and $\bar{\lambda}T$.

We are now in a position to summarize the steps to be taken in applying the sign method:

(i) By examining past records or by using preliminary observations from the trial itself, and consulting Table 7.2, estimate the value of λ for the standard treatment. Call this λ_0.

(ii) Estimate the rate of intake of subjects to the trial: m per unit time to each treatment.

(iii) From Table 7.3, calculate the expected number of preferences, G, obtained at various times, T, after the start of the trial. In this calculation $\bar{\lambda}$ is put equal to the value λ_0 estimated in (i). By interpolation calculate the values of T required to make G equal to various values of N corresponding to different restricted procedures (for example, those of Table 3.5).

(iv) To each of these values of N there corresponds a value of θ_1 which can be detected with high probability (see, for example, Table 3.5). Calculate $\lambda_B = 2\lambda_0 \theta_1$ and $\lambda_A = 2\lambda_0 (1 - \theta_1)$. Consult Table 7.2 for the proportions of survivors at various times after treatment for $\lambda = \lambda_A$ and $\lambda = \lambda_B$.

(v) In this way, one is able to see, for various values of T (which is an estimate of the maximum length of intake of patients), how big a difference between the survival curves one would have a good chance of detecting.

These considerations should provide a basis for the choice of a sequential design. It may be, of course, that a design is chosen with a particular value of N, and it is subsequently found that the initial estimates of λ_0 and m were so inaccurate that the time required to accumulate N preferences is very much longer or shorter than the value of T which was originally contemplated. To avoid this difficulty it would be wise to review the situation at an intermediate stage during the trial — not so much to compare λ_A and λ_B but to check the estimates of λ_0 and m. A revision of the sequential design might then be required.

It must be emphasized that the sign method provides a basis for a stopping-rule, but is not intended as a complete analysis of the data. If the sequential procedure leads to a decision to stop, one would naturally wish to follow the investigation, on the subjects already entered in the trial, so as to obtain more information about the survival curves. In the absence of any strong indication of the form of the survival curves the best procedure would probably be to analyse the data by life-table methods (see, for instance, the paper by Merrell and Shulman (1955)).

Example 7.1

In a trial to assess the efficacy of griseofulvin for the treatment of fungal infections, Russell *et al.* (1960) allotted patients randomly to groups receiving griseofulvin tablets or indistinguishable dummy tablets. The question was whether a "definite clinical improvement" occurred on the whole earlier in one treatment group than the other. The rate of occurrence of improvements was expected to be very low in the control group and it was thought that if the active drug was satisfactory, improvement might occur on the average in about three months. This would imply roughly that for griseofulvin $\lambda_B = 4$, for the control group $\lambda_A = 0$, and consequently $\bar{\lambda} = 2$ (time being measured in years). The estimated rate of entry was $m = 300$ pairs of patients per year. A practicable upper limit to the period of intake was 6 months, i.e. $T = \frac{1}{2}$ year. Thus $\bar{\lambda}T = 1$. From (7.2) and Table 7.2 (or by interpolation in Table 7.3), this implied $G = 150 \times 0\cdot57 = 85$. The restricted design with $\theta_1=0\cdot75$, $2\alpha = 0\cdot05$, $1 - \beta = 0\cdot95$, has $N = 62$, rather less than the value of G given above, but this was regarded as adequate for the purpose. Note that $\theta_1 = 0\cdot75$ implies $\lambda_B = 3\lambda_A$, a narrower difference than that considered above. An outer boundary was reached after 9 preferences had been recorded (all in favour of griseofulvin). The intake was stopped soon afterwards, when 76 patients had entered the trial. The follow-up continued until each patient had received the allotted treatment for 4 months. 12 patients did not complete the course of treatment. Of the remainder, 31 of the 33 patients treated with griseofulvin and only one out of 31 in the control group showed improvement during the 4 months' period.

A further example of the application of the sign method, using imaginary data, is described in detail by Armitage (1958b).

CHAPTER EIGHT

OTHER TYPES OF INVESTIGATION

8.1. Introduction

In the previous chapters we have considered the use of sequential analysis in trials in which treatments are compared simultaneously by random allocation. The importance of this method of conducting experiments has been stressed in Chapter 1. Certain other uses of sequential analysis in clinical medicine, although not falling under the heading of 'clinical trials' in this strict sense, are sufficiently close to the general topic of this book to warrant a brief mention.

8.2. Comparisons against a fixed standard

In some investigations a treatment may be evaluated against a fixed standard rather than by simultaneous comparison with another treatment. In view of the strong arguments in favour of randomization, cogent reasons must be provided before this important safeguard is abandoned. There are perhaps two main types of investigation in which the omission of randomization may be worth consideration.

(a) If only a few patients with the disease under study are available a comparison of two treatments by random allocation may be so insensitive as to be not worth doing. Suppose that extensive previous investigations provide a precise estimate of the effectiveness of one treatment (which may be referred to as the 'standard'), and suggest that this measure of effectiveness is fairly stable. If this stable level can be assumed to apply during the current investigation, all the available patients can be treated by the test treatment, and their responses compared with the assumed standard level. The precision of this comparison is equal to that in a randomized trial with four times as many observations; that is, the same precision is obtained with one-quarter the number of observations required in the randomized trial.

The difficulty is, of course, that the validity of the result depends upon the unverified assumption that the standard level is stable. The investigator may feel that in the circumstances it is better to have a reasonably precise comparison with a possibly doubtful standard, than a much less precise comparison with the safeguard provided by randomization. If he chooses this first course, though, it must be strongly emphasized that he has obtained a comparison between the response under the new treatment and a fixed level which he is willing to regard as being near the response of the standard treatment; he has *not* made a direct comparison of the two treatments.

(b) In the treatment of some diseases a large number of drugs may be available for trial. To submit each of these drugs to a full-scale clinical trial, with random allocation, may be impracticable with the resources available. A possible solution is to 'screen' the treatments by selecting only those which, in a pilot study, show sufficiently promising results. The successful candidates are then submitted to a proper clinical trial. Since authoritative and final judgment is not required in the pilot study, it will usually be adequate to compare the results from each treatment with a fixed standard. Treatments giving results clearly better than this critical level will be accepted quickly for further study. The much less effective treatments will quickly be rejected.

Sequential methods for making comparisons against fixed standards are described in the book by Wald (1947), and less mathematical expositions are contained in the books by the Statistical Research Group, Columbia University (1945) and by Davies (1954). Most of the plans described by these authors are open skew designs, for one-sided tests. Symmetrical designs for two-sided tests may be obtained by method (i) of Appendix A.2 of this book. Closed designs for many situations may be obtained by applying the results of Armitage (1957).

Detailed methods are not given here, because it seems unlikely that this sort of comparison will be frequently required. Examples of such investigations have been described by Doering *et al.* (1957), Hagans *et al.* (1957) and Johnson *et al.* (1959). It is not clear, from the accounts provided by these authors, whether their avoidance of random allocation was entirely justified.

8.3. Estimation procedures

A clinical trial conducted by the methods described in this book may stop so quickly, when the treatments differ much in effectiveness, that the extent of this difference cannot be estimated at all precisely. It is an unfortunate paradox that in just the circumstances when a difference is of most interest to the investigator he may be debarred for ethical reasons from measuring it accurately.

If there are no ethical difficulties the investigator should regard it as one of the main purposes of the trial to provide an accurate estimate of the difference in effectiveness between the treatments compared. In a non-sequential trial this accuracy will be determined by the number of observations made and the random variation which they show. The simplest type of sequential investigation has been discussed in §2.2 (b). If the random variation is not known initially, it may be estimated continuously as the observations are made, and the trial will be stopped when the estimated precision has been reduced to the required level. This precision is estimated by the standard statistical formulae.

This sort of investigation may be appropriate also for studies of differences between patients in different clinical categories in certain pathological tests. Vallee *et al.* (1956, 1957) have used sequential methods to study the levels of zinc concentration in normal subjects and in patients with different degrees of cirrhosis of the liver. They formulated their procedures as tests of particular hypotheses about the values of the differences between these groups. A more suitable approach would perhaps have been to estimate these differences with a specified degree of accuracy.

A different type of sequential estimation problem arises in studies of dose-response curves, where it is required to estimate the dose which corresponds to a particular mean response. The doses are varied from one observation to the next in such a way that they tend to concentrate around the required value. This type of procedure is strictly outside the terms of reference of this book, as defined in §2·1, since the treatment is deliberately varied throughout the investigation. The theory is incomplete at present, but these methods may play an important part in future research. Examples are the up-and-down method in biological assay (Dixon and Massey, 1957) and the Robbins-Munro method of stochastic approximation (Guttman and Guttman, 1959).

CHAPTER NINE

MISCONCEPTIONS AND DIFFICULTIES

9.1. Some misconceptions

(i) *Economy and significance.* The statement is sometimes made that a sequential analysis requires less observations than a non-sequential analysis because the investigation can be stopped as soon as a significant difference is detected. This assertion is misleading in more than one way. In the first place, we have observed in earlier chapters that if a sequential design is compared with a non-sequential design of the same power, the sequential design may be more economical *on the average*, but in a particular instance it may require more observations than did the non-sequential design.

Secondly, the statement carries the implication that the outer boundaries consists of points at which the difference is, in some sense, 'just significant'. To call a result significant at, say, the 5 per cent. level is to classify it among an extreme group of possible results which together will occur rather less than 5 per cent. of the time if the null hypothesis is true. If an attempt is made to attribute exact significance levels to particular boundary points, as in §3.5, inevitably some of these probability levels will be considerably below $0 \cdot 05$. It is nevertheless true that when large differences appear the investigation is stopped relatively early, and consequently results which are exceedingly improbable on the null hypothesis are avoided. For example, in the binomial designs considered in Chapter 3, the smallest values of P, calculated by the methods described in §3.5, are much greater than they would be in the equivalent non-sequential designs.

(ii) *Preliminary assumptions.* It is sometimes asserted that the setting-up of a sequential trial requires a preliminary guess at the results, and that the interpretation will be invalidated if this guess is inaccurate. This belief is quite fallacious. The quantities in terms of which a sequential design is defined, and by reference to which it is selected determine its power to detect a difference of a certain magnitude if this difference is present. The quantities θ_0 and θ_1, for instance, referred to in Chapter

3, are not guesses as to what the value of θ is likely to be, but represent differences regarded as so important that if they are really present the investigator will have a good chance of detecting them. It would be quite possible to classify non-sequential procedures in the same way, and indeed in choosing the sample size for a non-sequential investigation it is always advisable to consider the power function. As Cochran (1959) remarks:

'In the sequential trial, at the beginning, the doctor is forced to make some decisions about the desired sensitivity of the trial which he can dodge in the fixed-size trial. But to make an intelligent choice of the number of patients in a fixed-size trial, the same questions, or similar ones, must be answered. When sequential trials are better explained and better understood, they should not be any harder than fixed-size trials.'

9.2. Some difficulties

(i) *Change of boundaries*. Because the probabilities associated with a sequential design refer to a specified set of boundaries the investigator should make every attempt to follow the plan he has chosen. If he departs from the originally chosen design the interpretation of the results may be quite difficult.

The reasons for the departure may be unconnected with the observed differences between treatments. It may, for instance, be possible to follow a more powerful design than that originally intended, because more time is available or because more patients can be observed in the prescribed period. Conversely, the number of available patients may be less than had originally been estimated, and the design may have to be truncated sooner than had been intended. In either of these circumstances, a new design can be immediately applied and the results interpreted as though it had been the original choice. A change to a more powerful design may mean that observations continue beyond the original boundaries. A premature truncation will mean that a new inner boundary must be drawn. The theoretical properties of the amended plan may be difficult to work out, but the relevant probabilities can always be calculated exactly in trials involving series of preferences (Appendix A.4).

If the change of plan is decided on *because* of the observed difference the interpretation is much more difficult. It will usually not be possible to define precisely the new stopping-rule; and without a definite set of boundaries the probabilities cannot be calculated. One possible ap-

7§

proach would be to use standard non-sequential methods, and to realize that for the reasons stated in §1.7 the significance of departures from the null hypothesis is overstated. A more rigorous approach is to use the methods of subjective probability (see Appendix A.1) which have the merit of being entirely independent of stopping-rules, but provide no control over the 'error of the first kind' (the probability of mistakenly claiming a difference when in fact the null hypothesis is true).

(ii) *Combination of results.* How should one compare and combine results from different sequential experiments? There is no generally accepted solution of this problem. Perhaps the best advice is to form estimates of the appropriate means or proportions, with standard errors derived by standard non-sequential methods, and to compare and combine them by the usual large-sample methods. A rough justification for this suggestion is provided by the evidence mentioned in §3.6 that standard estimation procedures are not seriously invalidated by sequential experimentation.

A slightly different problem arises in a single sequential trial if a small number of observations are made after a boundary has been crossed. Usually the extra observations will be few in comparison with those made before the boundary was reached, and they will provide relatively little extra information. The essential result is then that given by the sequential analysis, and the extra results may be quoted without any attempt at quantitative combination. If the extra results are more numerous than those required by the sequential design the best solution is probably to analyse the whole collection of data by non-sequential methods, and to ignore the fact that a small proportion of the observations were made sequentially.

(iii) *The multivariate problem.* It was suggested in §2.4 (ii) that if the treatments are to be compared by a large number of response criteria, either those should be combined in some way or the trial should not be sequential.

The best way to combine a number of criteria in a sequential experiment is not known. In a non-sequential experiment, a possible approach is to form a discriminant function which combines the variables in such a way as to maximize the difference between the treatments in comparison to the random variation. It is not clear how this can be done in a sequential analysis, or even whether the result would be useful to the clinician, and the only possibility at the moment seems to be to determine the method of combination initially, perhaps by analysing previous results.

Suppose a sequential trial is performed on the basis of one variable,

x. How do we make comparisons on another variable, y, observed at the same time? If variations in x and y are quite unrelated, the results on y may be analysed by non-sequential methods. The fact that x was analysed sequentially does not in the least affect the interpretation of y. If y is very closely related to x, the non-sequential analysis of y will have much the same drawbacks as that of x — the significance of departures from the null hypothesis will tend to be overstated. In broad terms, y may be analysed by standard methods, but the degree to which the significance of departures from the null hypothesis is overstated will depend on the correlation between x and y.

(iv) *Interactions.* If the sequential analysis is carried out on pairs which are matched for various characteristics, it will be useful to know whether the difference in response between the two treatments varies from one stratum to another. For trials in which the treatments are compared within subjects, it might be asked whether the difference in response for the two treatments was greater for one type of subject than for another (e.g. whether it differs for the two sexes). In statistical terminology, the question is whether there is an *interaction* between the strata, into which the pairs are grouped, and the treatment effect. Cox (1960) has shown that if the paired observations are taken at random from the various strata (e.g. if males and females enter the trial in random order) these interactions may be investigated at the end of the trial by standard methods appropriate to non-sequential experiments. In the trial described in Example 3.3 the treatments were applied in random order. For the comparison of any two treatments, therefore, the subjects for whom treatment A preceded treatment B, and those who received B before A, formed a random sequence. The authors were therefore justified in applying a standard test (χ^2-test with continuity correction) to examine whether the proportion of preferences for A varied according to the order in which the treatments were applied. (Actually a restricted randomization, of the type described at the end of §2.5, was used, but this modification is unlikely to have much effect on the validity of the test.)

Order of administration is, of course, a factor which can be deliberately randomized. For factors like age, sex, severity of disease, the subjects will not follow one another in a strictly random order, but the order is likely to be sufficiently haphazard for Cox's result to be relevant. Rather more difficulty may be encountered in co-operative trials in which results are sent to a central point from various medical centres, and the question is whether the relative effect of the treatments varies from one centre to another. The results may be received from each centre in batches, so that the order is clearly non-random. Even here, if the results from the different centres are fairly well mixed in the sequential analysis, a standard type of test for the interaction of treatment and centre is unlikely to be seriously misleading.

(v) *The effect of various factors.* A slightly different question is whether various factors such as age, sex and severity affect the level of response (as distinct from the *difference* in response between treatments considered in (iv)). If the observations have been paired for the factor in question, the responses for each pair may be added, and a standard non-sequential analysis performed on these sums, at the end of the sequential experiment. If the observations are normally distributed the fact that a sequential analysis has been performed on the differences is entirely irrelevant to the analysis of the sums.

If the observations have not been paired for the relevant factor, the situation is less clear, but again it seems likely that a standard non-sequential analysis will be appropriate.

NOTES ON STATISTICAL THEORY

A.1. General

The procedures described in this book have been specified in terms of risks, the approach being that of Neyman and Pearson, and of Wald in his book on sequential analysis. Other suggestions for the specification of sequential stopping-rules have been made at various times. These include decision function procedures involving some quantitative assessment of the gains and losses incurred by following various courses of action. In contrast to this approach there are a number of alternative ways of indicating when the evidence against the null hypothesis is sufficiently strong for the experiment to be stopped. These include the use of likelihood ratios, with or without prior probabilities, and the application of information theory (Lindley, 1956). I have preferred to follow the Neyman-Pearson approach and to indicate in §1.5 that prior considerations and the consequences of courses of action should be taken into account, even though these factors are not expressed quantitatively.

It is, however, possible to consider briefly the interpretation of the sequential designs described in this book from the point of view of subjective probability (Savage, 1954). In a clinical trial the investigator will usually start with, at the best, slender evidence about the difference between the treatments to be compared. From the point of view of subjective probability this means that the prior probability distribution for the unknown parameter is not sharply peaked over the range considered possible, and a reasonable approximation might be to regard this prior distribution as uniform. It can then be shown, at least for normally distributed variables, that at any stage in the collection of observations, irrespective of the stopping-rule, the posterior probability that the parameter value is, say, less than zero, is exactly the same as the one-sided tail area of the usual *non-sequential* significance test of the null hypothesis that the value is zero. A similar result holds approximately for binomial observations. Now, when a sample path just reaches an outer boundary, in either the open or the closed designs described in this book, with a two-sided significance level 2α, the one-sided tail area probability in the orthodox non-sequential test is always less than α. It follows that, in the absence of any strong prior evidence, the posterior probability in favour of one treatment when an outer boundary is reached will be greater than $1 - \alpha$.

These considerations throw some light on the problem of the choice of boundaries. The designs described in this book have been chosen to satisfy two requirements; for example, in §3.3, the power is specified at $\theta = \frac{1}{2}$ and $\theta = \theta_1$ (the power at $\theta_0 (= 1 - \theta_1)$ being equal to that at θ_1 by symmetry). The boundaries used in Chapters 3–5 have, however, three arbitrary constants; for example, in §3.3, the constants a_1, a_2 and b. It follows that the sets of boundaries tabulated in these chapters are not unique (cf. Barnard, 1946, p. 10; Armitage, 1957, pp. 11–13). Why, then, are they advocated in preference to other possible boundaries?

In the first place, they are the simplest to obtain for any particular pair of requirements, being based on the likelihood ratio of the two hypotheses at which the power is specified (cf. §A.2). Secondly, the outer boundaries appear to be fairly satisfactory from the point of view of subjective probability. From the standpoint of subjective theory, it might be reasonable to stop taking observations, and to conclude that one treatment is better than the other, if the posterior probability that the difference parameter is positive (or the probability that it is negative) reaches a specified low value. As noted above, this will in practice be almost equivalent to performing repeated significance tests at some fixed level. The appropriate boundaries will clearly diverge but with an inward curvature. For example, in the situation discussed in Chapter 5, the equations of the outer boundaries would be

$$y = \pm k \sqrt{n},$$

where the constant k is determined by the critical posterior probability. These boundaries are not, of course, the same as those described in the earlier chapters, but the fact that they are divergent at least suggests that divergent linear boundaries are more acceptable than parallel or convergent ones.

One of the drawbacks of the subjective approach is that it provides no automatic check on the risks of coming to the wrong conclusions. As has been argued in §1.7, a danger of sequential experimentation is to increase the chance of claiming a difference in a specified direction when in fact none exists, and the methods described in this book provide a direct control of this risk. Perhaps the ideal state of affairs would be to use boundaries corresponding to a constant posterior probability, and at the same time to maintain a specified risk of rejecting falsely the null hypothesis. This reconciliation of the two approaches must await the solution of the relevant theoretical problems.

A.2. Two-sided open designs

Two alternative approaches have been made to the specification of two-sided open sequential tests (i.e. three-decision procedures), and as both of these approaches are used at different times in this book it may be useful to clarify the distinction.

Suppose a null hypothesis, H_0, is to be tested with two-sided error of the first kind (i.e. significance level) 2α; and that two alternative hypotheses, H_+ and H_- (symmetrically placed about H_0 in some sense), are to have errors of the second kind equal to β ($1 - \beta$ being the power of the test at H_+ and H_-). The three decisions favouring H_+, H_- and H_0 will be denoted by D_+, D_- and D_0. These correspond to the three conclusions (a), (a)' and (b) of §1.5. The two approaches are:

(i) To combine two Wald-type tests, T_+ which compares H_0 and H_+ with errors of the first and second kinds α and β, and T_- comparing H_0 and H_- with errors α and β; and

(ii) to compare H_0 with a composite hypothesis, giving equal weights to H_+ and H_-.

The method of combining T_+ and T_- in procedure (i) is indicated by the following table (Armitage, 1947; Sobel and Wald, 1949), showing the decisions to be taken in the combined test:

		Test T_+	
		Accept H_0	Accept H_+
Test T_-	Accept H_0	D_0	D_+
	Accept H_-	D_-	—

The fourth combination (accepting H_- and H_+) is precluded if α and β are both $<\frac{1}{2}$ and the likelihood function has no minimum. In procedure (ii) the alternatives are to accept or reject H_0, and in the latter case the distinction between D_+ and D_- is made by inspection of the data.

In most applications the two procedures will lead to similar stopping-rules for D_+ and D_-. For D_+, for instance, the stopping criterion under procedure (i) is

$$L_+/L_0 \geq (1 - \beta)/\alpha \qquad (A.1)$$

where L denotes the likelihood of the hypothesis indicated by the suffix. Under procedure (ii) the stopping criterion for D_+ is

$$(L_+ + L_-)/2L_0 \geq (1 - \beta)/2\alpha. \qquad (A.2)$$

In practice L_- will be negligible in comparison with L_+, and (A.1) will be very nearly the same as (A.2).

The stopping rules for D_0 will differ rather more. Under (i) the criterion is that L_0/L_+ and L_0/L_- shall both have exceeded $(1 - \alpha)/\beta$

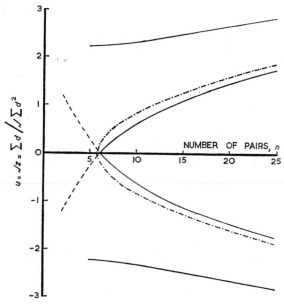

Fig. A.1. Two alternative open sequential t-tests with $2\alpha = 0\cdot05$, $1 - \beta = 0\cdot95$, $\delta_1 = 1$.

―――――― procedure (i); ― · ― · ― procedure (ii). (The outer boundaries for the two procedures are indistinguishable.)

at the present stage or some previous one. Under (ii), the criterion is that $2L_0/(L_+ + L_-)$ shall exceed $(1 - 2\alpha)/\beta$.

The interpretation of β differs a little in the two procedures. Under (i), β is the probability of taking D_0 or D_- when H_+ is true. Under (ii), β is the probability of taking D_0 alone. In either case the probability of taking D_- will be negligible in practice, and the distinction is unimportant.

As an illustration of the way in which the two types of procedure differ, Fig. A.1 shows the boundaries for two alternative sequential t-tests. The ordinate is $\sqrt{z} = \Sigma d/\sqrt{(\Sigma d^2)}$ (for notation, see §6.1), and the alternative hypotheses are $H_0 : \mu = 0$; $H_+ : \mu = \sigma$, $H_- : \mu = -\sigma$, with $2a = \beta = 0\cdot05$. For procedure (i), two skew designs with $a = 0\cdot025$, $\beta = 0\cdot05$ are used. Details of these are given by Rushton (1950), and the combined test is described by Davies (1954). The boundaries were obtained by interpolation in Davies's Table L.5, for $a = 0\cdot025$, $\beta = 0\cdot05$, or by fresh computation. For procedure (ii), the boundaries tabulated in the N.B.S. tables (see §6.2) are adapted by plotting the square root of the boundary point and preserving the sign of Σd. It is theoretically possible (but very unlikely) under procedure (ii) to jump from one channel to the other without taking decision D_0, whereas under (i) such a jump would imply that the boundary for D_0 had been crossed. The rather closer approach to the origin by the D_0 boundary, under (ii) as compared to (i), is counter-balanced by the possibility under (i) of taking D_0 when both dotted lines have been crossed.

It is fairly clear that the two approaches will usually lead to very similar results, and there is no strong reason other than that of convenience for choosing one rather than the other. In this book procedures of type (i) are used for binomial observations (Chapter 3) and for normally distributed observations with known variance (Chapter 5), because they lead to linear boundaries. For normally distributed observations with known variance the procedure of type (i) is a particular case of that described by Sobel and Wald (1949); the corresponding procedure of type (ii) is given by Wald (1947) and described further by the Statistical Research Group, Columbia University (1945). The sequential t-test described in Chapter 6 is a type (ii) procedure, and is advocated here because of the extensive tabulation in the N.B.S. tables. The corresponding type (i) procedure is described and tabulated by Davies (1954).

A.3. Two-sided closed designs

The 'restricted' procedures of Armitage (1957) are formed by using the same boundaries for D_+ and D_- as were required by open procedures of type (i), and, for linear boundaries, determining the 'cut-off' value, N, by an approximation based on diffusion theory. Further theoretical results are given in an important paper by Anderson (1960). Since these outer boundaries, leading to decisions D_+ and D_-, differ very little from those for the corresponding procedures of type (ii), the same value of N could be used as an approximation for both types of procedure. The values of N for the non-linear sequential t-test are obtained by further and more conjectural approximation (see §6.3).

A.4. Computations for binomial designs

With any sequential design for a binomial series of preferences, such as those tabulated in Chapter 3, the probability of reaching each boundary point may be calculated exactly as a function of θ (the probability of a preference for treatment A). The probability of reaching a boundary point at which there have been r preferences for A, and $n - r$ for B, is

$$\nu \theta^r (1 - \theta)^{n-r},$$

where ν is the number of ways of ordering the preferences in such a way that no boundary point is reached at a previous stage. In the visual representation used in Chapter 3, ν is the number of accessible paths to the boundary point in question, i.e. paths which avoid previous boundary points.

The evaluation of ν is the main problem. This is best done by evaluating the numbers of paths to points *between* the boundaries for successively increasing values of n. Simple matrix multiplication facilitates the calculations. For details see Stockman and Armitage (1946).

Exact calculations of this type were used for the entries in Tables 3.7–3.10, and for the smaller designs specified in Tables 3.5 and 3.6. In Tables 3.1 and 3.2 the coefficients defining the boundaries are obtained from the well-known formulae of Wald, appropriate for one-sided tests with two parallel boundaries.

The entries in columns (b) and (c) of Tables 3.1 and 3.2 are obtained from the formulae given by Wald for the one-sided test. For some of the smaller designs, some sampling experiments and the application of the formula given by de Boer (1953, p. 254) suggested that the entry in column (a) of Table 3.1 should be approximately mid-way between those in columns (b) and (c). This approximation was therefore used in Table 3.1. Approximate values for the entries in column (a) of Table 3.2 were obtained by slight adjustment to those in Table 3.1 (the inner boundaries for corresponding designs in the two tables being very similar).

REFERENCES

ANDERSON, T. W. (1960). A modification of the sequential probability ratio test to reduce the sample size. *Ann. math. Statist.*, **31**, 165–97.

ANSCOMBE, F. J. (1954). Fixed-sample-size analysis of sequential observations. *Biometrics*, **10**, 89–100.

ARMITAGE, P. (1947). Some sequential tests of Student's hypothesis. *J. R. statist. Soc. Suppl.*, **9**, 250–63.

ARMITAGE, P. (1954). Sequential tests in prophylactic and therapeutic trials. *Quart. J. Med.*, **23**, 255–74.

ARMITAGE, P. (1957). Restricted sequential procedures. *Biometrika*, **44**, 9–26.

ARMITAGE, P. (1958a). Numerical studies in the sequential estimation of a binomial parameter. *Biometrika*, **45**, 1–15.

ARMITAGE, P. (1958b). Sequential methods in clinical trials. *Am. J. publ. Hlth.*, **48**, 1395–1402.

ARMITAGE, P. (1959). The comparison of survival rates. *J.R. statist. Soc.*, A, **122**, 279–92.

ARMITAGE, P. and HEALY, M. J. R. (1957). Interpretation of χ^2 tests. *Biometrics*, **13**, 113–5.

BAILEY, N. T. J. (1959). *Statistical methods in biology.* London: English Universities Press.

BARNARD, G. A. (1946). Sequential tests in industrial statistics. *J.R. statist. Soc. Suppl.*, **8**, 1–21.

BILLEWICZ, W. Z. (1956). Matched pairs in sequential trials for significance of a difference between proportions. *Biometrics*, **12**, 283–300.

BILLEWICZ, W. Z. (1958). Some practical problems in a sequential medical trial. *Bull. Inst. int. Statist.*, **36** (3), 165–71.

BILLEWICZ, W. Z. (1959). Use of sequential analysis in a clinical trial. In *Quantitative methods in human pharmacology and therapeutics.* Edit. D. R. Laurence. London: Pergamon Press.

BROSS, I. (1952). Sequential medical plans. *Biometrics*, **8**, 188–205.

BROSS, I. (1958). Sequential clinical trials. *J. chron. Dis.*, **8**, 349–65.

COCHRAN, W. G. (1950). The comparison of percentages in matched samples. *Biometrika*, **37**, 256–66.

COCHRAN, W. G. (1959). Newer statistical methods. In *Quantitative methods in human pharmacology and therapeutics.* Edit. D. R. Laurence. London: Pergamon Press.

COCHRAN, W. G. and COX, G. M. (1957). *Experimental designs.* 2nd ed. New York: Wiley.

COX, D. R. (1958a). *Planning of experiments.* New York: Wiley.

COX, D. R. (1958b). Two further applications of a model for binary regression. *Biometrika*, **45**, 562–5.

COX, D. R. (1960). A note on tests of homogeneity applied after sequential sampling. *J. R. statist. Soc.*, B, **22** (in the press).

DAVIES, O. L. (Edit.) (1954). *Design and analysis of industrial experiments.* London and Edinburgh: Oliver & Boyd.

DE BOER, J. (1953). Sequential test with three possible decisions for testing an unknown probability. *Appl. Sci. Res.*, B, **3**, 249–59.

DIXON, W. J. and MASSEY, F. J. (1957). *Introduction to statistical analysis.* New York: McGraw-Hill.

DOERING, C. R., HAGANS, J. A., ASHLEY, F. W., CLARK, M. L. and WOLF, S. (1957). Sequential analysis in therapeutic research. I. Application to binomial data and to measured data normally distributed (one-sided alternative). *J. Lab. clin. Med.*, **50**, 621–8.

ENDICOTT, K. M. (1957). The chemotherapy program. *J. nat. Cancer Inst.*, **19**, 275–93.

FISHER, R. A. and YATES, F. (1957). *Statistical tables for biological, agricultural and medical research.* 5th ed. Edinburgh and London: Oliver & Boyd.

FLAVELL MATTS, S. G. (1960). Local treatment of ulcerative colitis with prednisolone-21-phosphate enemata. *Lancet*, i, 517–9.

FLETCHER, C. M. and OLDHAM, P. D. (1959). Diagnosis in group research. In *Medical surveys and clinical trials.* Edit. L. J. Witts. London: Oxford University Press.

GUTTMAN, L. and GUTTMAN, R. (1959). An illustration of the use of stochastic approximation. *Biometrics*, **15**, 551–9.

HAGANS, J. A., DOERING, C. R., CLARK, M. L., SCHNEIDER, E. M., and WOLF, S. (1957). Sequential analysis in therapeutic research. II. Application to measured data normally distributed (two-sided alternative). *J. Lab. clin. Med.*, **50**, 629–38.

HAJNAL, J., SHARP, J. and POPERT, A. J. (1959). A method for testing analgesics in rheumatoid arthritis using a sequential procedure. *Ann. rheum. Dis.*, **18**, 189–206.

HILL, A. B. (1951). The clinical trial. *Brit. med. Bull.*, **7**, 278–82.

HILL, A. B. (1956). *Principles of medical statistics.* 6th ed. London: Lancet.

HILL, A. B. (1960). (Edit). *Controlled clinical trials.* Oxford: Blackwell.

JOHNSON, E. A., HAUS, E., HALBERG, F. and WADSWORTH, G. L. (1959). Graphic monitoring of seizure incidence changes in epileptic patients. *Minn. Med.*, **42**, 1250–7.

KILPATRICK, G. S. and OLDHAM, P. D. (1954). Calcium chloride and adrenaline as bronchial dilators compared by sequential analysis. *Brit. med. J.*, ii, 1388–91.

LINDLEY, D. V. (1956). On a measure of the information provided by an experiment. *Ann. math. Statist.*, **27**, 986–1005.

MCNEMAR, Q. (1949). *Psychological statistics.* New York: Wiley.

MAINLAND, D., HERRERA, L. and SUTCLIFFE, M. I. (1956). *Tables for use with binomial samples.* New York University College of Medicine.

MARSHALL, J. and SHAW, D. A. (1960). Anticoagulant therapy in acute cerebro-vascular accidents. *Lancet*, i, 995–8.

MEDICAL RESEARCH COUNCIL. (1948). Streptomycin treatment of pulmonary tuberculosis. *Brit. med. J.*, ii, 769–82.

MEDICAL RESEARCH COUNCIL. (1955). Various combinations of isoniazid with streptomycin or with P.A.S. in the treatment of pulmonary tuberculosis. *Brit. med. J.*, i, 435–45.

MEDICAL RESEARCH COUNCIL. (1956). B.C.G. and vole bacillus vaccines in the prevention of tuberculosis in adolescents. *Brit. med. J.*, i, 413–27.

MEDICAL RESEARCH COUNCIL. (1957). The assessment of the British vaccine against poliomyelitis. *Brit. med. J.*, i, 1271–7.

MEDICAL RESEARCH COUNCIL. (1959). Vaccination against whooping cough. *Brit. med. J.*, i, 994–1000.

MEIER, P., FREE, S. M. and JACKSON, G. L. (1958). Reconsideration of methodology in studies of pain relief. *Biometrics*, **14**, 330–42.

MERRELL, M. and SHULMAN, L. E. (1955). Determination of prognosis in chronic disease, illustrated by systemic lupus erythematosus. *J. chron. Dis.*, **1**, 12–32.

MORONEY, M. J. (1956). *Facts from figures.* 3rd ed. Penguin.

NATIONAL BUREAU OF STANDARDS. (1951). Tables to facilitate sequential *t*-tests. (Applied Mathematics Series, 7.) Washington: U.S. Dept. of Commerce.

NEWTON, D. R. L. and TANNER, J. M. (1956). *N*-acetyl-para-aminophenol as an analgesic. A controlled clinical trial using the method of sequential analysis. *Brit. med. J.*, ii, 1096–9.

POLIOMYELITIS VACCINE EVALUATION CENTER. (1955). *Evaluation of 1954 field trial of poliomyelitis vaccine.* Ann Arbor: The National Foundation for Infantile Paralysis. (Summary report in *Am. J. publ. Hlth.*, 45, No. 5, Pt. 2.)

ROBERTSON, J. D. and ARMITAGE, P. (1959). Report of a clinical trial to compare two hypotensive agents. *Anaesthesia*, 14, 53–64.

RUSHTON, S. (1950). On a sequential *t*-test. *Biometrika*, 37, 326–33.

RUSHTON, S. (1952). On a two-sided sequential *t*-test. *Biometrika*, 39, 302–8.

RUSSELL, B., FRAIN-BELL, W., STEVENSON, C. J., RIDDELL, R. W., DJAVAHISZWILI, N. and MORRISON, S. L. (1960). Chronic ringworm infection of the skin and nails treated by griseofulvin. *Lancet*, i, 1141–7.

SAINSBURY, P. and LUCAS, C. J. (1959). Sequential methods applied to the study of prochlorperazine. *Brit. med. J.*, ii, 737–40.

SAVAGE, L. J. (1954). *The foundations of statistics.* New York: Wiley.

SMITH, J. MORRISON. (1958). Hydrocortisone hemisuccinate by inhalation in children with asthma. *Lancet*, ii, 1248–50.

SNELL, E. S. and ARMITAGE, P. (1957). Clinical comparison of diamorphine and pholcodine as cough suppressants, by a new method of sequential analysis. *Lancet*, i, 860–2.

SOBEL, M. and WALD, A. (1949). A sequential decision procedure for choosing one of three hypotheses concerning the unknown mean of a normal distribution. *Ann. math. Statist.*, 20, 502–22.

STATISTICAL RESEARCH GROUP, COLUMBIA UNIVERSITY. (1945). *Sequential analysis of statistical data: applications.* New York: Columbia University Press.

STOCKMAN, C. M. and ARMITAGE, P. (1946). Some properties of closed sequential schemes. *J. R. statist. Soc. Suppl.*, 8, 104–12.

THOMSON, T. J. (1958). Clinical comparison of methyprylone and quinalbarbitone as hypnotics. *Brit. med. J.*, ii, 1140–1.

TRUELOVE, S. C. (1958). Treatment of ulcerative colitis with local hydrocortisone hemisuccinate sodium. A report on a controlled therapeutic trial. *Brit. med. J.*, ii, 1072–7.

VALLEE, B. L., WACKER, W. E. C., BARTHOLOMEY, A. F. and ROBIN, E. D. (1956). Zinc metabolism in hepatic dysfunction. I. Serum zinc concentrations in Laënnec's cirrhosis and their validation by sequential analysis. *New Engl. J. Med.*, 255, 403–8.

VALLEE, B. L., WACKER, W. E. C., BARTHOLOMEY, A. F. and HOCH, F. L. (1957). Zinc metabolism in hepatic dysfunction. II. Correlation of metabolic patterns with biochemical findings. *New Engl. J. Med.*, 257, 1055–65.

VAN EEDEN, C. (1955). A sequential test with three possible decisions for comparing two unknown probabilities, based on groups of observations. *Rev. Inst. int. Stat.*, 23, 20–28.

WALD, A. (1947). *Sequential analysis.* New York: Wiley.

WATKINSON, G. (1958). Treatment of ulcerative colitis with topical hydrocortisone hemisuccinate sodium. A controlled trial employing restricted sequential analysis. *Brit. med. J.*, ii, 1077–82.

WITTS, L. J. (1959). (Edit.) *Medical surveys and clinical trials.* London: Oxford University Press.

INDEX

AUTHOR INDEX

SUBJECT INDEX